M000207109

7 Ways to Transform the Lives of Wounded Students

7 Ways to Transform the Lives of Wounded Students provides a wealth of strategies and ideas for teachers and principals who work with wounded students—those who are beyond the point of "at risk" and have experienced trauma in their lives. Sharing stories and examples from real schools and students, this inspirational book examines the seven key strategies necessary for changing school culture to transform the lives of individual students. Recognizing the power of effective leadership and empathy in creating a sense of community and safety for wounded students, Hendershott offers a valuable resource to help educators redesign their school environment to meet the needs of children and empower educators to direct students on a path to academic and life success.

Joe Hendershott has an extensive background as an educator and administrator in private, public, and higher education. He is the founder and president of Hope 4 The Wounded, LLC, an educational consulting business.

Other Eye on Education Books Available from Routledge

(www.routledge.com/eyeoneducation)

Reaching the Wounded Student
Joe Hendershott

Five Critical Leadership Practices:
The Secret to High-Performing Schools
Ruth C. Ash and Pat H. Hodge

Mentoring is a Verb: Strategies for Improving
College and Career Readiness
Russ Olwell

How to Make Data Work:
A Guide for Educational Leaders
Jenny Grant Rankin

A School Leader's Guide to Implementing
the Common Core:
Inclusive Practices for All Students
Gloria D. Campbell-Whatley, David M. Dunaway, and
Dawson R. Hancock

Hiring the Best Staff for Your School: How to Use
Narrative to Improve Your Recruiting Process
Rick Jetter

What Connected Educators Do Differently
Todd Whitaker, Jeffrey Zoul, and Jimmy Casas

BRAVO Principal! Building Relationships with
Actions that Value Others, 2nd Edition
Sandra Harris

Creating Safe Schools:
A Guide for School Leaders, Teachers,
Counselors, and Parents
Franklin P. Schargel

7 Ways to Transform the Lives of Wounded Students

Joe Hendershott

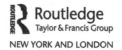
Routledge
Taylor & Francis Group

NEW YORK AND LONDON

First published 2016
by Routledge
711 Third Avenue, New York, NY 10017

and by Routledge
2 Park Square, Milton Park, Abingdon, Oxon, OX14 4RN

*Routledge is an imprint of the Taylor & Francis Group,
an informa business*

© 2016 Taylor & Francis

The right of Joe Hendershott to be identified as author of this work has been asserted by them in accordance with sections 77 and 78 of the Copyright, Designs and Patents Act 1988.

All rights reserved. The purchase of this copyright material confers the right on the purchasing institution to photocopy or download pages which bear the eResources icon and a copyright line at the bottom of the page. No other parts of this book may be reprinted or reproduced or utilized in any form or by any electronic, mechanical, or other means, now known or hereafter invented, including photocopying and recording, or in any information storage or retrieval system, without permission in writing from the publishers.

Trademark notice: Product or corporate names may be trademarks or registered trademarks, and are used only for identification and explanation without intent to infringe.

Library of Congress Cataloging-in-Publication Data
Names: Hendershott, Joe, author.
Title: 7 ways to transform the lives of wounded students /
    Joe Hendershott. Other titles: Seven ways to transform the
    lives of wounded students
Description: New York, NY : Routledge, 2016. | Includes
    bibliographical references.
Identifiers: LCCN 2015034359 | ISBN 9780415734943 (hardback) |
    ISBN 9780415734950 (pbk.) | ISBN 9781315819501 (ebook)
Subjects: LCSH: Children with mental disabilities—Education. |
    Abused children—Education. | Post-traumatic stress
    disorder in children—Treatment.
Classification: LCC LC4601 .H39 2016 | DDC 371.9—dc23
LC record available at http://lccn.loc.gov/2015034359

ISBN: 978-0-415-73494-3 (hbk)
ISBN: 978-0-415-73495-0 (pbk)
ISBN: 978-1-315-81950-1 (ebk)

Typeset in Palatino
by Apex CoVantage, LLC

For my children: Kaelee, Kearsten, Kameryn, Kyler, Kade, K'Tyo, Kaya, Kemeri, and Kendi. Being your father is an honor and a privilege, and I love each of you for who you are. Every one of you inspires me to do better and love bigger. 'Ohana.

Contents

Acknowledgments

With special thanks:

To my wife, Dardi, it's special to walk this journey alongside of you. There are no words to adequately describe the love, support, and dedication you have given to me during this project. None of this would be possible without you. I love you.

To Dr. Terry Wardle, thank you for sharing your knowledge and heart for working with wounded people. What I have learned from you is foundational to the work that I do.

To Dr. Harold Wilson, thank you for your support as a mentor, adviser, and friend.

To Dr. Greg Gerrick, thank you for being a constant source of encouragement in my endeavors. Great teachers never quit cheering on their students.

To Ken Packard, I appreciate your insights based on your experiences and research that you have always been willing to share. I am grateful for you.

To Dr. Constance Savage, I appreciate the way you challenged me to keep my focus on the learning, and then to be a good steward of that knowledge.

To my editor, Heather Jarrow, thank you for your patience and encouragement along this journey.

Preface

On November 23, 2012, we laid my father to rest. Despite the frigid temperature and it being the day after Thanksgiving, we were overwhelmed by an enormous outpouring of people who came to the church to pay their respects. Envision a very large church sanctuary with people lined up from the front all the way back to the narthex and around through a receiving line of family for over three straight hours before the service. I had never seen many of these people before in my life, but each expressed sentiments similar to, "Your dad made a difference in my life." One man looked me in the eye and said, "Your dad saved my life."

My dad was not a doctor, a therapist, a lawyer, or a teacher. He was a recovering alcoholic. For anyone who understands addiction, being an overcomer of that addiction could be a legacy in and of itself. My dad enjoyed the quiet of his cabin in the woods and could have easily spent his many years of sobriety in the sanctuary of that peaceful existence but instead, he became a source of hope, encouragement, and accountability to those in the trenches of addiction. He recognized their pain and was willing to be a part of their transformation, many times at the expense of his own personal comfort.

There are wounded people everywhere in the world, and as educators, our scope of influence is great. We have the opportunity to connect with others on a daily basis. Some of those relationships are easy to cultivate, but some involve a level of investment that can be challenging and even messy. The wounded students in our schools find themselves struggling to climb their way out of the ditch, much like the people that crossed paths with my dad. What I have determined in my life is that people are more receptive to help out of the ditch if I am willing to stand with them at the bottom, understanding that the climb out is going to be rough. If I only know the view from the top of the ditch, my advice for getting out is not going to bear much weight and may even come across as judgmental and callous.

It is my belief that most people go into education with the desire to share their passions and abilities with the next generation. Much of our teacher preparation is based on the delivering of knowledge; unfortunately, the fact that the path to some children's learning is marred with obstacles is not given the same level of emphasis. At the time of my father's passing, I was a student myself in the midst of the most stressful aspect of my doctoral work. My 86-year-old professor and doctoral adviser, Dr. Harold Wilson, was present at the funeral and in the coming days as I had to navigate rigorous coursework in the midst of my grief. It is because of his empathy and unwavering belief in me that I found the strength and courage to keep going in my studies. Do not underestimate your connection with your students, regardless of their age.

Who Is This Book For?

This book is designed specifically for anyone in the educational arena (school board members, superintendents, central office administrators, building administrators, teachers, school counselors, school nurses, support personnel, etc.). The focus is about how we can all play a part in helping to transform the lives of the wounded children that cross our paths. We all serve in a caregiver capacity, so to understand our students at a deeper level allows us to utilize teachable moments to deeply impact their lives.

However, I would also suggest that the content of this book is suitable for anyone working with wounded children, be it parents, foster/adoptive parents, YMCA employees, youth pastors, youth camp counselors, businesses that employ students, or juvenile court judges—and the list goes on. There are many people who find themselves involved in the lives of wounded children, but who don't necessarily have any familiarity or ongoing support for understanding the effects of trauma on their lives and how to work with them.

It is my hope that anyone looking to understand and feel empowered to work with wounded children will be able to share in my 30+ years of experience as both a foster/adoptive parent and as an educator who has served in the positions of administrator and teacher in a multitude of settings including correctional and alternative education. In addition to sharing from my firsthand experiences, I have researched the topic from experts and turned to professionals in the mental health and medical fields to further enhance my own understanding as well as that of you, the reader.

Organization of the Book

This book begins with the idea that we need leaders when it comes to how we work with the wounded children in our schools. The more leaders, or agents of change, that we have, the better chance wounded students have at finding success. Once your leadership potential is recognized, the next chapter looks at trauma and the effects it can have on everything from identity and behavior to the learning process itself. Trauma has a significantly negative impact on a child's development and thought processes, which is why the third chapter delves into the way we need to consider the whole brain in learning and interactions, especially with wounded children.

Moving into the fourth chapter, the discussion moves to emotional literacy, most specifically the need for empathy. How do we connect with students who are coming from hard places that many of us cannot even fathom? Not only do we need to make empathic connections with students, but we need to position them to give and receive empathy to/from others. This encourages an emotionally safer learning environment and can reduce instances of bullying.

Empathy is also a critical first step in building a sense of community. Community is essential in helping wounded children feel connected to something bigger than themselves. To go from feeling isolated or rejected to being a valuable member of their school and local community is transformational. Everyone needs to have a sense of belonging and purpose.

The final two chapters will give the reader some takeaway strategies for professional and personal consideration. The nine professional checkpoints in the sixth chapter focus on what we can do to encourage the process of transformation in the lives of the wounded students we encounter. Both individual and group approaches are discussed to promote safety, security, self-esteem, and establishing meaningful connections with wounded students. The final chapter includes nine checkpoints for taking care of ourselves and our inner learner. Knowing ourselves, our needs, our strengths, and our areas of weakness is an ongoing journey in life. By not periodically taking a look inward, we can drastically reduce our ability to continually give outward, which is contrary to why we became educators in the first place.

Let's Get Started

My good friend and mentor, Dr. Terry Wardle, told me once that it's not about guilt, it's about vision. It is my hope that in the pages of this book, you find inspiration for reigniting your original motivation for becoming an educator, a better understanding of the challenges you face, a vision for yourself and your students, and the encouragement to be the difference that brings transformation to the lives of wounded people. Many of us have known the struggle of trying to find hope in dark places and are thankful for the people who have stepped into our lives to assist in finding hope. As my father demonstrated, those areas of greatest weakness can evolve into a wounded student's area of greatest strength through the help of people who connect with the student, displaying compassion and empathy. One day, they will look back and remember those who helped transform their broken lives as they walk forward with a sense of purpose and hope.

Meet the Author

Joe Hendershott is a graduate of The Ohio State University. He earned his Doctor of Education in educational leadership studies and holds a Master's Degree in school administration from Ashland University, and he is currently an administrator in higher education. Joe also has an extensive background working with difficult and troubled youth in the school system. He has been a high school assistant principal, head principal, alternative school principal, and principal at Boys' Village School (residential treatment facility).

As president of his own consulting firm, Hope 4 The Wounded, LLC, Joe has presented at national educational conferences and has conducted staff training/professional development on understanding and working with wounded students, emotional literacy, empathy, esteem, inclusive communities, and other topics relevant to today's educational climate. His workshops are designed to equip, empower, and encourage those who endeavor to discover and cultivate the unique abilities and gifts that all children possess.

Introduction

This book has been a work in progress for several years, and quite frankly, there were many times that it felt like it would never come to fruition. Family, the demands of my job, the rigors of being enrolled in a doctoral program as well as time constraints in general were certainly contributing factors to the lengthy process, but even more perplexing was the fact that this whole concept of learning how to work with wounded students is a complex matter. I have spent many years trying to explain the difference between students deemed "at risk" and the students I consider to be wounded.

At-risk students are typically identified based on certain situational criteria including, but not limited to, socioeconomic factors, family composition, physical or learning disabilities, English as a second language, truancy, and/or low performances on tests. Many different studies have been done on the at-risk student population, but these seem to be the most common risk factors used in identifying those students deemed at risk of not graduating high school.

On the other hand, I define wounded students *as children who have experienced or continue to experience emotional and/or physical traumatic events. This has a profound impact on their physical, emotional, and/or spiritual identity as well as their ability to function in the classroom and in life.* There are certainly similarities between at-risk and wounded students, but interventions for the at-risk population of students are usually based on risk factors making the student susceptible to negative outcomes.

In contrast, interventions for wounded students begin with the awareness that these children are not in in danger of something happening to them; something *has happened* to them. They have crossed over from being at risk to being a casualty of their circumstances. For many wounded students, that very trauma becomes the lens through which they view every person and circumstance. As educators, we must acknowledge that wounded students have already experienced trauma, develop an understanding of the impact of trauma on a child's brain function, and become intentional with the way we seek to connect with and accommodate these students to give them the best chance at making it.

Over the last several years, many educators have begun making, and even embracing, the distinction between at-risk and wounded students. While this is encouraging, I have still struggled with trying to emphasize enough that the need for education and training specific to working with wounded students is imperative on a national scale. There is a plethora of literature available geared towards the at-risk student population, which is fantastic. There is also a wealth of information about childhood trauma, brain development, and emotional literacy; but I have been looking for that connection that would validate my experience and research about the vital need for educators to have access to well-rounded training involving all of these critical components so they are equipped to deal with the trauma that is walking through their doors every day.

I have come to believe that timing is everything, and sometimes there is a reason that things like this book do not come together as quickly as we would like them to. In March of 2015, I submitted the bare bones of the manuscript I had been working on the past several years and then began the task of edits and additions in April and May. On May 21, 2015, my wife sent me a link to an article dated May 18, 2015 entitled, "Landmark Lawsuit Filed in California to Make Trauma-Informed Practices Mandatory for All Public Schools" (Paull, 2015). And there it was . . . the link I and so many other educators, parents, and caregivers have made and have been passionate about for years was finally being recognized as a very real problem. According to the article, "A landmark first step was taken today to insure that all public schools in the United States be legally required to address the unique learning needs of children affected by adverse childhood experiences" (Paull, 2015, p. 1). The article further stated that the legal team is basing its case on the research findings that have established that adverse childhood experiences (ACEs) are obstructing the ability of millions of children to succeed in school. According to Paull:

> "ACEs" comes from the CDC-Kaiser Adverse Childhood Experiences Study (http://www.cdd/gov/violencepre vention/acestudy/), a groundbreaking public health study that discovered that childhood trauma leads to the adult onset of chronic diseases, depression and other mental illness, violence, and being a victim of violence. The 10 ACEs the researchers measured include physical, sexual and verbal abuse, physical and emotional neglect, a family member who is depressed or diagnosed with other mental illness, addicted to alcohol or another substance, in prison, witnessing a mother being abused, losing a parent to separation, divorce or other reason.
>
> (2015, p. 2)

Mark Rosenbaum, directing attorney for Public Counsel's Opportunity Under Law Project, is quoted as saying, "Childhood trauma is the number one public health problem in the U.S. today." I am encouraged by the fact that more people are acknowledging the need to better prepare educators to work with wounded students in a way that provides transformational interventions instead of only utilizing strategies that are punitive in nature. I believe the recognition of this need can most certainly prove to be advantageous to not only the children, but also those who have been entrusted with providing their education and care as well as communities as a whole.

By establishing the very real need for trauma-informed practices, my hope is that the suggestions contained in these pages and the referencing of relevant research act as a catalyst for ongoing research and training on the topic; but it cannot end there. Even greater than the knowing is the doing, otherwise known as *stewardship*. As defined on Dictionary.com (n.d.), stewardship is "the responsible overseeing and protection of something considered worth caring for and preserving." Educators tend to feel that deep sense of responsibility towards their students, but the reality of walking in that stewardship can be challenging. If we can equip ourselves in order to remain focused on stewardship, we can not only reach our wounded students but also begin the journey of transformation in their lives. Galford and Seibold Drapeau (2002) discuss this in the context of one's legacy, stating, "a winning legacy might be framed in terms of business accomplishment: organizational growth, geographic expansion, survival or salvation. For others, legacy has to do with more of a stewardship role, where their legacy is one of keeping the asset going, and handing it over to a new generation" (p. 230). Sergiovanni further stated:

> Students are not clients, customers, or cases, but objects of stewardship. Stewardship requires that adults have a personal stake in the academic success and the social welfare of each student. Stewardship requires that adults bring a collective orientation rather than self-orientation to bear in their relationships to students and with each other, placing the common good over their own personal interests.
>
> (1994, p. 102)

Embracing a concept of a legacy of stewardship is important because it allows us as educators to focus more on the big picture of what we are trying to accomplish in our careers. It involves not only how we impact the present, but also the possibilities for transformation of the future. Anyone can easily become complacent and caught up in the mundanities of day-to-day operations, so it is meaningful to view things from a legacy perspective. In my first book *Reaching the Wounded Student,* I developed a model—which can be found on page 15 of that book—for reaching wounded students based on my beliefs, observations, firsthand experiences as an educator, and research up to that point, which may help people to remain focused on the big picture. I believe this model still holds true, with the addition of one final piece: Transformation. According to Merriam-Webster.com, to transform something means to change it completely, and usually in a good way. Wounded students have experienced trauma that disconnects them from finding academic and life success. Our goal needs to be to reconnect them and get them back on track, which will lead to transformation in their lives. The model is as follows:

The Hendershott Model for Reaching the Wounded Student

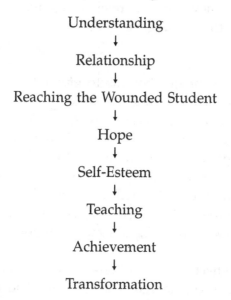

Understanding
↓
Relationship
↓
Reaching the Wounded Student
↓
Hope
↓
Self-Esteem
↓
Teaching
↓
Achievement
↓
Transformation

In order to institute trauma-informed practices, one must first develop an understanding of the effects of trauma. Once there is awareness and understanding, healthy relationships can be cultivated with sensitivity. Through this relationship, you have established an avenue for reaching the wounded student, which in turn acts as an anchor of hope, increasing self-esteem. All of this is foundational so that teaching, and therefore achievement, can commence. This achievement leads to wounded students becoming victors over their adversity, which is transformational to their lives. With regard to transformational experiences among survivors of trauma, Jaffe (1985) said, "Their whole feeling about themselves changes as [they release feelings of pain, self-pity, anger, or helplessness.] They feel qualitatively different, without denying or forgetting the wounds they have experienced" (p. 107). Jaffe further stated:

> When there is a realization on a conscious or unconscious level that transformation has taken place, a transformation forged in the fire of their adversity and pain, survivors may perceive positive meanings in their ordeals. Their adversity now becomes the cornerstone of a new identity, as they now discover a positive meaning or message in their struggle or pain.
>
> (1985, p. 107)

My intention for this book is to give educators an understanding and some inspiration for working on a daily basis with children who have experienced brokenness. While they are not with us 365 days a year, our wounded students are never far from our thoughts. It is easy to let our thoughts wonder where they are, how they are doing, whether they are safe, whether they have food and shelter, will they even be able to come to school? Sometimes, just seeing a wounded student walk through the door to school is the biggest victory we can hope for on any given day.

As I have reflected on the different thoughts I have had over the years, I have considered what I wish I had known along the way to better serve this marginalized population of students. It is in this spirit that I wanted to author this book, to benefit aspiring educators as well as those already in the trenches. It is the culmination of many years of experience, my own successes and failures, as well as research from experts in the fields of brain research, emotional intelligence, and the effects of trauma. In my own journey as an educator seeking to reach every student coming into my classroom or office, I felt like gaining information on these topics was a bit of a hunt and peck endeavor. My hope is that this book is just the beginning of a conversation in which we acknowledge the need for trauma-informed practices; a meeting place for an array of information supported by research that can positively impact our work with children of trauma in the classroom.

This book is not a one-size-fits-all guide to putting the pieces of the puzzle together, but inspiration for putting peace into the lives of wounded students so they can truly begin to experience success in learning. This is where transformation begins. Transformation is an ongoing process for everyone. Do you feel you are a different person now than you were twenty years ago? Do you expect that you might be somewhat different twenty years from now? You will hear this from me often: What is true of them is true of me, and what is true of me is true of them.

This book is also not designed to fix or control broken kids or merely survive their presence in our classrooms. It is not a guarantee that transformation will happen within a day, a month, a year, or ever. It is about how certain principles can apply to all of us as we seek to build relationships with wounded children to meet their social, emotional, and academic needs, which is vital to positioning students for transformation.

This book begins with an appreciation for how we can all be leaders in working with wounded youth. Just by being educators, we are put into the position of being first responders in the lives of wounded children, so I will propose different avenues for stepping into that leadership/first responder role. As a first or front-line responder, it becomes necessary to know how to identify trauma and recognize the effects that trauma can have on everything from the brain to behaviors to learning. It is within these chapters that you will find some incredible research findings from experts in the fields of trauma, brain development, and emotional literacy.

Research to support the need for empathic connections will also be shared. A compassionate, empathic community plays a major role in positioning wounded students for transformation by mitigating stressful responses with feelings of safety and security that are conducive to learning and academic achievement.

In the final two chapters, I chose to leave you with professional and personal strategies to consider as educators committed to providing hope for all students. Some of them may be new ways of thinking, while others may have been fundamental in your journey. Whatever the case may be, it is always good to have some checkpoints for consideration when investing so much of your heart and soul into your students. When you are in the thick of challenging behaviors or seeing hopelessness in ways you never thought possible, it is good to be encouraged to tap into your own inner strength, abilities, and gifts to keep pressing forward to make a difference. I can honestly say that it is worth it, as I have had the privilege of witnessing so many broken lives transformed into strong, contributing members of their families and communities. Their own hardships became their biggest strengths, which resonates with my own journey thus far. What is true of them is true of me, and what is true of me is true of them.

We cannot change the past for wounded students, but we can strive to make the changes necessary to positively impact their futures. My challenge to educators is to take your scholarship and integrate it with your heart, imagining what the future could be. Bring that vision to life as you seek to bring transformation to the lives of your wounded students. They need you, and I believe in you.

> "Being courageous requires no exceptional qualifications, no magic formula, no special combination of time, place and circumstance. It is an opportunity that sooner or later is presented to us all."
>
> —John F. Kennedy, Thirty-Fifth President

1

Become a Leader

Where to Begin

Truth be told, I struggled with where to begin this book. There are seven important aspects to transforming the lives of wounded students, and my original intent was to place the topic of leadership at the end as a way of sewing the first six points together. However, I kept coming back to the reality that leadership is where transformation starts. Who is going to step up as an example for positioning students to experience transformation in their lives? We must first have people who recognize the need is great in order to begin the "doing."

I have been asked by educators on numerous occasions, "What is it that these students must do to turn their lives around? What skills must they develop to be successful?" I would like for us to begin a new conversation by asking the questions in a different way: "What can *I* do to help turn students' lives around? What skills can *I* develop to be successful in helping my students?" This is where leadership begins.

Early in my career, I sought that person who was going to provide leadership and an example of what to do with these struggling kids. What I usually found was frustrated professionals, up to and including myself, who had more questions than answers. At some point, the realization came that if I felt it was important to have an impact on the lives of wounded students, then I needed to be willing to step into a leadership role by seeking knowledge and creative pathways to opportunities for transformation in their lives.

Educators today can feel isolated within their content or area, so the idea of leadership can be daunting. My personal experience of developing as a leader in working with wounded students did not come easily. Any unfamiliar territory that we venture into may be challenging and even intimidating, feeling like an area of weakness instead of an avenue for growth and potential. Robert Louis Stevenson once said, "You cannot run away from weakness; you must some time fight it out or perish; and if that be so, why not now, and where you stand?" The realization came that if I was going to be effective as a teacher, and eventually as a school administrator, I was going to have to take the plunge and develop my inexperience into an intentional awareness, because there were often wounded students in my classrooms.

I encourage you as an educator—be it teacher, counselor, or administrator—to look at what leadership capacity you have in regard to understanding wounded students, so that you can identify areas for development. I believe it is imperative that everyone within an organization should see themselves and others as an integral part of the whole picture, taking a broader view of the educational team and its efforts to reach every member of its student population, including the wounded students. Kouzes and Posner observed, "Trust is the social glue that binds human relationships" (2006, p. 71), and Thompson further stated, "We cannot study leadership by isolating people and their behaviors from the social-organizational settings in which they act" (2008, p. 180). As members of a team, it is fair to have the expectation of receiving professional training that extends a systems view, forcing team members to work together to better service all children.

How to Begin

First, understand that you do not have to become a counselor, therapist, psychiatrist, or other mental health specialist to be a leader working with wounded children. I do not hold any of these certifications or degrees myself, but over the years I have aspired to deepen my capacity as an educator to understand wounded children. In the pages of this book, you will find various strategies for working with wounded children as well as an understanding of the effects of trauma. However, just as we are constantly seeking effective methods for teaching subject matter, I always encourage schools to continue in their pursuit of ideas for and understanding of wounded children through ongoing professional development. So, where does professional training come from that can provide understanding and equip us for working with wounded students? One excellent resource is the local social services agency. Typically, they are more than happy to provide professional training and insight on working with children from traumatic backgrounds. Another valuable resource can be your local law enforcement officers. They have had specialized training in deescalating situations, which is an integral part of keeping students in the classroom. Additionally, pediatricians, mental health professionals, and child development specialists can provide invaluable information about how traumatic experiences affect brain development, esteem, learning, and behaviors. As a school leader, one of my biggest areas of personal growth was the recognition of the need for well-rounded training for myself and my colleagues, addressing the real challenges facing educators working with children of trauma who are struggling behaviorally, socially, and/or emotionally, in order to help them discover their full potential. There is still a tendency towards hesitation, fear, or uncertainty when we start questioning the school policies, handbooks, and discipline guidelines that have been the normal way of doing things for a long time, and this is understandable. However, the wounded children in our schools fall outside the textbook practices many guidelines are built upon. We need leaders to rise up to challenge these norms using current research as well as personal experiences, so that the need for training beyond preparation to work with only the traditional student population is recognized.

privacy rights

Famous National Football League and Hall of Fame Coach Vince Lombardi once said, "Contrary to the opinion of many people, leaders are not born. Leaders are made by effort and hard work." The willingness to take a leadership role in bringing transformation to the lives of wounded students is definitely hard work. It requires positioning others as well as yourself to be prepared to understand the students who are hurting the most. That very understanding expresses itself as sincerity, which wounded students are very adept at perceiving. Positioning ourselves to understand can lead to wounded children being more open to receiving help, guidance, instruction, and encouragement.

What Are You Trying to Change?

Effective leadership in bringing about transformation or change for wounded students should begin with three questions. First, *what* are we trying to change? Many answers will be unique to the challenges facing your particular school culture, so I would suggest doing a survey to determine if there is a consensus among team members about what they see as the most necessary changes. Of course, we always strive for academic achievement, but I believe that will naturally occur when we are seeking ways to develop our students as individuals in that process.

Some possibilities for change might include suspension rates, graduation/dropout rates, attendance rates, or maybe something as simple as creating a better sense of community for children and faculty alike.

At this juncture, I would like to share that I have had instances where the overwhelming response as to what needs to be changed was student behavior. This kneejerk reaction is totally understandable, but this is where reflection on the part of the educator is helpful. When working with wounded children, it is almost a given that some types of dysfunctional behaviors are involved. The whole point of trying to bring about transformation in wounded students' lives is to find a way to see past the behaviors to find hope in a child, instead of trying to control behaviors or take them personally. When wounded children begin to feel the hope that we see in them, their behaviors will naturally begin to evolve. In many instances, assistant principals or guidance counselors have been the only team members who have had any instruction in this kind of response to dysfunctional behaviors. Again, professional training will enable a universal understanding of wounded children and their behaviors as well as encouragement for developing consistent, productive avenues of response to those behaviors.

Dr. Martin Luther King, Jr. surmised:

> The arc of the moral universe is long, but it bends towards justice. Social justice to me should start with the children in our schools. This is where they should understand that we have an equal playing field and that their hopes and dreams can be realized during these formative years.

Dr. King was the epitome of an ethical leader. According to Brown and Trevino, ethical leaders do not just talk a good game. They practice what they preach and are proactive role models for ethical conduct (2006). Dr. King recognized that schools are a place to reach all children, and he believed in the change he was preaching.

What do you think needs to change? Do you believe in it enough to become an ethical leader for that change?

Who Are You Trying to Change?

The second question that needs to be asked is *who* are you trying to change? Do you seek to evolve as an educator in regard to your approach to working with wounded children, or are you maintaining your current approach with the expectation that the wounded student will change? What would be the answer for your school as a whole?

If we are trying to change ourselves to meet the needs of wounded youth, then we need to be honest about where we are in that process. Identifying areas that are proving to be difficult helps us to make effective choices when requesting types of professional training. As more and more educators take steps into becoming leaders who communicate specific needs as a team, those requests will show consensus toward a common goal. As Goleman said, "Leadership is not about domination, but the art of persuading people towards a common goal" (2006, p. 149).

If the expectation is that wounded students will change to conform to traditional approaches, the hill becomes steep and everyone will struggle. I know change is hard, I do. And change is harder for some than for others, and it does not happen overnight. This is where leadership matters, and some leadership happens through action rather than words.

Several years ago, I was invited to provide professional development for a school district in Ohio. The woman who had orchestrated the training had previously heard me speak at a conference. She was totally on board with making changes to bring transformation for wounded students and had put into practice many of the ideas I had shared. A few years later, I heard back from her. She shared that in the beginning, the training was not well received by many staff members. However, over time, and having witnessed transformation happening for some students, many of those same staff members chose to become active agents of change in their school. (You will find a more detailed letter from Julie about this school's experience later, in Chapter 7.) Gandhi said it best when he said, "Be the change that you wish to see in this world."

Why Are We Trying to Change?

Finally, we need to ask *why* are we trying to change? According to recent statistics from the National Center for Educational Statistics, U.S. Department of Education, the graduation rate was 80% for the school year 2011–2012 (Stetser & Stillwell, 2014). This percentage of graduates approaches a forty-year high in the United States. I don't know about you, but if I received an 80%

on anything in high school, I was doing cartwheels around the block. Just me? Well, at any rate, 80% seems pretty okay. Or is it?

- ◆ 80% of a graduating class of 400 = 320 graduates, 80 non-graduates
- ◆ 80% of a classroom of 20 = 16 graduates, 4 non-graduates
- ◆ 80% of a lunch table of 5. . . . Yes, one of those 5 kids is not going to make it.

It is easy to get lost in big numbers, but when you break it down to actual faces in your school, in your classroom, or a child at the lunch table, these numbers are just not okay.

Educators are by nature caring and giving individuals who want the best for all their students. Sometimes it is difficult to rise to that task or just easier to look to others to lead the way for change. Northouse said, "Leadership is a process whereby an individual influences a group of individuals to achieve a common goal" (2007, p. 3). There is a pressing need for change, and for leaders to step up in our schools in order to spearhead that change. Wounded students need people who look very much like you.

"If your actions inspire others to dream more, learn more, do more and become more, you are a leader."

—*John Quincy Adams*

The Big Picture

Chapter 1
Key Points

♦ Everyone within an organization should see themselves and others as an integral part of the whole picture, with everyone willing to step into a leadership role to reach every member of the student population.

♦ Every person in the school organization is in a position to be a transformational leader in the developmental years of a child's life.

♦ It takes commitment, desire, and ongoing training to become a leader in reaching wounded children.

♦ Seek professional development opportunities specific to working with children from traumatic backgrounds.

♦ Asking who, what, and why we are trying to change gives focus to your personal and organizational mission. The motivation for change should always be transforming the lives of wounded children.

2

Recognize the Effects of Trauma

"Although the world is full of suffering, it is full also of the overcoming of it."
—Helen Keller

Before I get into the thick of this chapter, I want you to understand that my point of reference is not solely based on my experiences and research as a professional practitioner. I am also a parent to children who experienced trauma early in their lives before coming into our family. There is sometimes a misconception that wounded children are a product of their current environment, and so it is easy to place blame on their home life for the struggles you see in the classroom. You might be surprised to find many parents who would love nothing more than to team up with you in an effort to help their child. And as the parent of wounded children, my passion for empowering and equipping practitioners with understanding and tools for working with these children runs deep, as my own growth and understanding has come to a very personal level over the last few years.

While there is plentiful research about at-risk children and how to set up programs to assist them, the current dilemma involves what to do with *traumatized* youth in our schools and communities. Oftentimes in schools today, we try to treat our wounded students as at-risk students, resulting in unsuccessful outcomes. Children who are wounded need a different level of understanding for us to have successful outcomes in and out of the classroom. This chapter will draw on the expertise of several theorists and specialists with regard to understanding trauma and its overall effect on the learning process. Gleaning insights from this type of information is imperative to bringing transformation into students' lives. Moreover, the importance of training is supported by the fact that "one out of every four children attending school has been exposed to a traumatic event that can affect learning and/or behavior" (The National Child Traumatic Stress Network, 2008, p. 4).

At this point, I would like to emphasize that recognizing trauma in your students, seeking interventions for a student in crisis, and making accommodations for the wounded students in your classroom does NOT in any way suggest that you are the one responsible for providing therapy or healing. Much like someone who has witnessed an accident where a child has broken his/her arm, unless you are a trained medical provider with the proper equipment on hand to set that broken arm, you will initially take on the role of first responder. Your job at that point is to acknowledge the situation, call emergency personnel (trained professionals), and provide reassurance and compassion until professional help arrives. Being an educator, healing a broken arm is out of your area of expertise, but you can still be a first responder. Not only can you be a first responder, but you can also be willing to walk alongside your student as they recover. You cannot hurry your student's healing along, but you can be sensitive to the fact that their healing journey may need accommodations and grace along the way.

In the case of a child coming into school with a broken arm, which also happens to be the hand they write with, you would most certainly be empathic to that limitation and even become inventive with modifying some things to make your student's daily work more manageable. So it is with wounded children. Over the years, I have witnessed the pain and struggle of many students on their quest for healing. It took time and a great deal of patience with themselves and others, but the road to healing and transformation tends to be smoother for students who find themselves in a culture of understanding, compassion, and empathy. If students are in cultures that only have pockets of understanding, compassion, and empathy, the healing process can be interrupted and the road to healing becomes more difficult and frustrating, sometimes even detouring into further dysfunctional behaviors if the student continues to feel misunderstood, judged, or isolated by those around him.

Understanding Wounds

To better understand wounded students, Dr. Terry Wardle (2007), a leading expert in the field of trauma and wounded behavior, discussed the causes and effects of wounds, including:

♦ *Wounds of withholding*: When a child's physical and/or emotional needs are not met by their caregiver.
♦ *Wounds of aggression*: When a caregiver has acted in a physically and/or emotionally abusive way toward a child.
♦ *Wounds of stressful events*: When an uninvited event happens that is beyond what is considered normal in a child's life.
♦ *Wounds of betrayal*: When a caregiver misuses or abuses power with a child.
♦ *Wounds of long-term duress*: When a prolonged season of pressure or pain has a devastating effect on a child/person.

According to Wardle, the typical cycle of wounds is as follows:

1. *Wound*: When a traumatic event leaves a deep impact on a person's life experience.
2. *False beliefs*: The wound stirs up negative feelings in a person, which leaves them in an uncomfortable state.
3. *Emotional upheaval*: The wound and false beliefs can lead to sadness, depression, shame, or other unsettled feelings.
4. *Dysfunctional behavior*: This occurs when people respond to their pain in negative, unhealthy ways.
5. *Life situations*: This is when the wound creates distortions or disorders that override even the original event (2007, p. 103).

Fallout from Trauma

Viewing trauma through the lens of a fight, flight, or freeze response gives a sharpened sense of the body's reaction to a traumatic event. Think of instances where students in your care have suddenly lashed out in anger at you or another student, have had a meltdown over something seemingly minor, have become withdrawn or fixated on fiddling with an object, have stared off into space, not responding to directions given, and so forth. At first glance, these behaviors present as misbehavior or noncompliance, and you might be wondering what this has to do with the wounds children already had coming into your classroom. Research suggests that unresolved trauma can manifest itself as post traumatic stress disorder. The implication is that trauma plays a role in our overall wellbeing (Scaer, 2005), and it can affect both our emotional and physical health. According to O'Neill, Guenette, and Kitchenham (2010), most current research supports the notion that early childhood traumatic experiences affect one's lifelong learning. It is further suggested that teachers and school counselors would understand trauma responses from children better if they were provided with proper training on what they can expect from children of trauma. Those behaviors mentioned above? It could very well be that they had absolutely nothing to do with the child's desire to behave or be respectful but were actually a response to a trigger bringing back feelings associated with previous trauma.

Children may or may not have control over certain emotional or social behaviors in the classroom. Since trauma can be hidden, it is difficult for people outside of the immediate family or caregiver situation to properly recognize the behaviors that accompany trauma. Typically, these behaviors are labeled as unacceptable in today's school cultures. They can be viewed as laziness, carelessness, low cognitive function, or refusal to participate in daily class activities. They can also be misconstrued as Attention Deficit Hyperactive Disorder (ADHD), Oppositional Defiant Disorder (ODD), an anxiety disorder, or depression (Tishelman, Haney, O'Brien, & Blaustein, 2010). In some instances, behaviors can be manipulative in nature, disguised as charm or affection. These are learned behaviors, developed when children find themselves in situations where they are trying to survive and struggle to trust that their core needs will be met.

Educators can struggle to identify traumatized youth because traumatic events sometimes happen in isolation. For instance, violence in families is not widely known or discussed outside the home, and so identifying victims of family violence can be difficult for teachers or staff members (Tishelman, Haney, O'Brien, & Blaustein, 2010). Another illustration comes from my personal experience as an adoptive parent. Most adoptive parents today speak openly about their children being adopted. However, we tend to be very protective regarding the circumstances that led to our children needing to be adopted, out of respect for our children. The personal details of their stories are theirs. The best advice I have for educators is that sometimes the most important thing to understand about trauma is that even though we may never fully understand it, it is critical that we seek to recognize children of trauma and implement interventions.

Trauma Interventions

One specific intervention that has been identified is the need for bullying prevention. Bullying prevention and intervention play vital roles in helping to protect wounded children, as well as keeping students from experiencing trauma at an early age. Victims of bullying typically suffer from physical symptoms including sleep issues, depression, thoughts of suicide, and anxiety. These students could also have low self-esteem and other issues with their overall emotional health (Vreeman & Carroll, 2007). Because wounded students sometimes exhibit some of these symptoms, their behavior may be misunderstood as being rooted in their traumatic background rather than in the bullying that has compounded their difficulties. Vigilance in awareness of the dynamics of peer interactions and creating safe environments is essential to bullying prevention. Creating safe communities in our schools is discussed further in Chapter 5.

Another research-proven intervention program, developed by Little, Akin-Little, and Gutierrez, is Trauma-Focused Cognitive Behavior Therapy (TF-CBT). TF-CBT has six core values (Little, Akin-Little, & Gutierrez, 2009):

1. *Meets individual needs*: No rigid, step-by-step approaches.
2. *Respect*: Be sensitive to religious beliefs, community, and culture.
3. *Adaptability*: Be flexible and creative with each individual.
4. *Family involvement*: Utilize family or caregivers to assist with designing intervention.
5. *Therapeutic relationship based on trust and empathy*: Modeled by therapist or counselor and adhered to by all involved parties.
6. *Self-efficacy*: This is the ultimate goal for the individual/ family for functioning after intervention.

Jaycox, Langly, Stein, Wong, Sharma, Scott, and Schonlau (2009) studied a positive intervention pilot program called Cognitive Behavioral Intervention for Trauma in Schools (CBITS), and the initial results show positive outcomes for this program, used by teachers and school counselors. Some of the cognitive behavioral interventions that have proven beneficial for students include:

1. *Psycho-education*: Develop an understanding of how students may react to trauma.
2. *Training on relaxation techniques*: Serves to calm down the student triggered by trauma.
3. *Cognitive coping*: A productive way of expressing feelings or thoughts.
4. *Mastery of trauma*: An understanding of the effects of trauma enables one to assist students in a competent way.
5. *Processing traumatic memories*: Use media or first-person recollections as resources for the details of the trauma.
6. *Social problem-solving*: Practice critical-thinking skills in a group of peers or adults in order to find solutions for difficulties.

I am sure you have already seen the distress caused by standardized testing and the increased expectations placed on students and teachers alike in regard to some academic standards. In the midst of all the demands, I urge you to continue to be mindful of ways to celebrate the uniqueness of our individuality—yours included—which cannot be measured by a test. This mindfulness will help as you face the reality that trauma walks through the school doors every day within the souls of too many children. Judging trauma, pitying trauma, or blaming trauma does not deal with trauma. The only way to deal with trauma is to acknowledge it and try to understand how it may be affecting a child's behaviors and learning. That's where the transformation will begin.

"Trauma is a fact of life. It does not, however, have to be a life sentence. Not only can trauma be healed, but with appropriate guidance and support, it can be transformative."

—*Peter A. Levine*

Chapter 2
Key Points

- One out of every four children has experienced trauma.
- The first step in bringing transformation into a wounded child's life is an understanding of the effect trauma has on attitudes, behaviors, and ultimately, learning.
- Typologies of wounds:
  1. Withholding
  2. Aggression
  3. Stressful vents
  4. Betrayal
  5. Long-term duress.
- Effects of wounds:
  1. Wounds
  2. False beliefs
  3. Emotional upheaval
  4. Dysfunctional behavior
  5. Life situations.
- Trauma affects emotional and physical health.
- The road to transformation is smoother for wounded students when they are immersed in a compassionate and empathic culture.
- Having trauma intervention programs in place is beneficial when crises occur.

3

Include the Whole Brain

Last year, I gave presentations to over 3500 educators from across the country in Nashville, Tennessee, at the largest high school conference in the country. With regard to wounded students, I asked how many of them felt they had a basic level of knowledge for dealing with the wounds that some of their students were coming into school with. I prefaced this by saying that I was not asking about psychiatrist-, psychologist-, social worker-, or counselor-level knowledge, but about a *basic* level of knowledge. Only two educators raised their hands. In order to effectively gain an understanding of wounded students, we need to have a basic understanding of how the brain works.

The Left Brain

Most educators have been schooled at universities that approach learning from a left-brain perspective, i.e. from the perspective of the cognitive part of the brain. Many educators have been successful as students and become teachers because this mode of learning worked for them. Once in the classroom, the right-brain model of learning is not typically considered, because what is measured on state and national exams is based on left-brain learning. As we seek to transform the lives of wounded students, I believe one of the first steps is to understand how integrating both hemispheres of the brain is not only beneficial, but is also a necessary approach to relationships, problem solving, and thinking.

The left part of the brain serves a very distinct purpose and can be of great benefit to problem solving and critical thinking. The ability to organize thoughts and think critically is an essential skill set as we travel through life. However, problems arise when we utilize only our left brain when a situation, such as understanding wounded students, requires us to think in a more abstract, emotional, or right-brained manner.

Siegel and Bryson refer to the left and right brains as having a mind of their own. They operate from two very different places, and both have a function that can clearly complement the other when fully integrated. The left brain is responsive to things that are logical, literal, and linguistic, and likes things that are linear, sequenced, and ordered (Siegel & Bryson, 2011).

It is helpful to understand that the left brain is very rule driven. It is not uncommon for educators to seek rules and guidelines to be followed in their teaching strategies as well as their schools. This is a very natural left-brain strategy for ensuring a sense of direction and order for our students. However, problems arise when the rules and guidelines become absolutes in a world where we need the ability to understand that not every circumstance can be approached from a left-brain perspective. Certainly, there are times when it is vital to follow the letter of the law. For example, in the instance of physical safety, total compliance is non-negotiable. However, I have found over the years that many situations we face as educators fall in a gray area. When working with children and making decisions regarding them, there tend to be extenuating circumstances to take into consideration. It is easy to give a rigid response in an effort to make sense of a situation or try to control the chaos surrounding it, but issuing wounded children with logical advice or consequences without first listening to their story can trigger further confusion and chaos. What happens to the student struggling with depression and suicidal thoughts? Or the student who has just been removed from his/her home and placed in foster care? Their behavior may be such that we would be well within our rights to demand their removal from our classrooms or even our schools, but if we consider these particular circumstances, isolating these students would be devastating to their emotional wellbeing. The left brain says that rules are rules. However, we need to acknowledge that every child brings their story to school, and that this requires a more empathic, right brain response. This may be very contrary to the way some of us were raised or trained, but a one-size-fits-all mentality when it comes to expectations and consequences just does not work with wounded children. If we fail to factor in students' cultures and sub-cultures and recognize their differences, we will not be serving our students well and will be discounting their disparities (Wardle, 2011).

If your tendency is to operate from a left-brain perspective, hear me when I say that I am not being critical of you. Being more of a left-brain person can also serve as an advantage, as long as we recognize how the brain operates and how to use its unique capabilities to most effectively meet the needs of those around us. If we have a student who is emotional and very much in the right-brain mode, it is best to listen and attune to what the child is saying: the *connect and redirect approach* (Siegel & Bryson, 2011). In an effort to keep the situation from escalating by trying to move too quickly from right- to left-brain processing, a good strategy is to ask "what" questions. This opens the door to the child telling their story, which helps them put their emotions in order and feel like they are being heard. Once connected and calm, the situation is more conducive to logical thinking. Contrarily, asking "why" questions (or even "what" in an accusatory or sarcastic tone) immediately sends children into a defensive mode, which only leads them further away from logical thinking.

I once heard someone say that modeling is the purest form of teaching, and I believe this to be true. Thus far, I have addressed the left-brained thinking from an educator's perspective because it is very difficult to get students to become whole-brain thinkers if we are not willing to take on this approach ourselves. Most schools are designed for the left-brain student, which is referenced in my first book with the 1/3 Model. School norms work well for the top 1/3 of the students who are able to "set and get." Included in that 1/3 are children who are well-adjusted, both mentally and emotionally, who abide by the letter of the law and who tend to be rule oriented themselves. When these children enter school, they can focus on academics, follow rules, and have the ability to connect easily with teachers and others. Many of these children can engage in the left-brain material given to them by teachers, thinking rationally and analyzing the information given. We reinforce this tendency toward strict adherence when we say things like, "The teacher is always right," or "Do what you are told and you will be fine." Though at their core these are very good notions when it comes to behavior, they do not assist in developing a whole-brain child and can put wounded children on the defensive, since trauma forces functioning in a very opposite capacity to left-brain logical thinking.

The Right Brain

While we need to teach children to be respectful to the thoughts, feelings, and position held by their teachers, we also want to encourage the critical and creative thinking that asks questions and seeks answers outside of the box. In an era of high stakes testing and goal-minded curriculum being at the forefront of education, it can be very difficult for teachers to apply much of the whole-brain concept to instruction. The idea of integration is being lost. According to Siegel (2007), "The right hemisphere is better at seeing context and the whole picture than the more detail oriented left hemisphere" (p. 45). We are not teaching our children to see the whole picture—nor are we considering the whole picture of a child—when we teach them all the same way and measure them without considering other factors that play into their young lives. If children develop the attitude that they should just go through life doing what they are told and take on the beliefs of another as absolute, we are bound to become a society that is robotic and lacking innovation.

The right brain is totally separate from the left brain in how it serves our needs. The right side of the brain picks up on nonverbal cues such as eye contact, facial expressions, posture, tone, and gestures. It manages our memories and our emotions

(Siegel & Bryson, 2011). The right brain is also concerned with feelings and relationships. It is the creative or artistic part of our brain and can respond to activities such as music, dance, or even sports. In addition, the right side of the brain is very holistic, and pays attention to body sensations. Our emotional and social being is housed in the right hemisphere of the brain, as well. It is the site of our primitive emotions (Wardle, 2011).

It is important to understand how people function in the right brain. I would like to highlight a few areas that can become a problem in today's schools and classrooms for students who function primarily in right-brain mode. If a right-brain student seldom prioritizes, this fundamentally goes against how the educational system operates. Based on the current standards, the state outlines what should be taught, when, and to what level. The teachers, in turn, give out syllabuses so students can set up their schedules, do their homework, and then be neatly prepared for the big test. This works well for left-brain students, but right-brain students may get lost in the face of the require-ment for strong prioritization, organizational, and time manage-ment skills. The other possibility is that a right-brain learner may not even read the directions at the beginning of the semester since they may be more of an auditory learner. It is important for educators not only to understand these differences, but also to be equipped to handle them. It is all too easy for teachers to get frustrated with this type of student, because they challenge the norms. Right-brain learners will probably do well in classes such as art or music, where their creativity is not only expected, but appreciated. The problem is that due to our lack of under-standing of the whole-brain child and the overall importance subjects such as art and music hold for brain development, these programs are being cut back or eliminated. The reasoning is that it will allow more time for students to study measured content areas such as math, science, or social studies. However, many people who study the importance of retaining the arts as part of the educational experience support the notion of whole-brain learning. "If educational processes in schools, colleges, and graduate and professional programs like medical school leave out one mode or the other, the integration needed for balanced learning will be absent" (Siegel, 2007, p. 235). This point should be stressed to school policymakers as they start eliminating programs that would benefit everyone's whole-brain learning. Programs such as music, art, or media are classes that evoke feelings in a person. Things like finger painting or holding objects provide sensory input and feelings (Wardle, 2011).

When conducting professional development or speaking at a conference, I often ask attendees to think back through their own academic careers and their teachers along the way. People will use an emotional connector or a right-brained feeling response, whether positive or negative, when a teacher's name comes up. I almost never hear a left-brain response like, "He was a great teacher of fractions," or "She really understood physics." I hear responses such as, "He was cool and made me feel good," or "She was so positive." At the other end of the spectrum, I might hear, "He never smiled," or "She was a grouch and didn't like kids." I have had instances where people actually break down and cry when reflecting on a teacher because the emotional connection is so strong. This exercise is designed to try to create a positive neuropathway; to create a positive neuropathway by drawing on a defined point of reference from their personal experiences (Wardle, 2011). These memories are stored in the right brain. When giving opportunities for doing right-brain activities with students, it is always good to make them feel safe and let them share what they are feeling with the group if they want to. It may be the first time they have processed their right-brain thoughts and feelings.

The right brain may also be the part of our brain that saves us with a fight or flight response. When we are in imminent danger, the last thing we want to do is go to our left brain and cognitively think about the danger and then decide methodically how to respond. By the time we have sorted it out, it could be too late for our own personal safety. Logic does not serve a purpose for the fight or flight response (Scaer, 2005).

The right part of the brain is very social, so it is important in our classrooms that we do not just lecture and teach without providing opportunities for interaction. Many of my college students who have taken the opportunity to teach overseas share that the biggest difference they see in other countries is that there is not so much competition in the classrooms. Many of the teachers use group work, which fosters critical thinking and social skills.

Another ability of the right brain is to have empathy or attune to others. Siegel and Bryson stated, "The art of considering the mind of another requires us to use our right hemisphere and upstairs brain" (2011, p. 137). Having this type of understanding about how to reach students who are wounded is vital if we are going to be effective teachers and administrators. Many of our schools have policies and procedures that exclude or isolate students when they bring their dysfunctional behavior to the school. School leaders tend to take the left-brain approach when dealing with behaviors, which is very ineffective. Taking time and connecting with that wounded child and developing a relationship is a right-brain modality. I feel that as a school leader, it is critical to get staff to look past the behavior and try to find the redeeming quality of that student. By finding something good to focus on, we meet students at their current level and can begin to understand why the behavior might exist. As mentioned before, taking the time to connect and know a child's story helps us to deescalate a situation because we are letting the student know that they are not about to be isolated in a room or out of school.

As educators, we should strive for our students to be empathic with each other, and if they are more empathic, there should be fewer instances of bullying. Empathic relationships could have a major impact on our schools becoming more emotionally safe for everyone. If we want this to take place, we must model this empathic, right-brained approach in our school rules and consequences. Empathy must be considered at all levels if we are going to help our wounded students feel included and heal on an emotional level, which usually does not happen from the left-brain, cognitive level. Programs like peer mediation can help students learn how to develop problem-solving skills through empathic approaches. It allows them to practice this skill and then remain in school if they can solve their own conflicts.

Another aspect of looking at the right brain and our discipline policies is that we need to make students feel like we understand them. When dealing with behaviors, we need to make sure students feel like they still belong and provide them hope through our positive feedback. This will make them feel safe, and it also lets the student know we have time for them. We need to stop processing students' behaviors through a system of suspensions and expulsions and then expect them to respond differently the next time they become emotional or upset.

The left part of the brain can serve as part of the healing and learning process as it can help make sense of the world around us and make us feel safe and secure. The key is to understand when it can be detrimental, since we must be able to use this part to connect to the right side for total integration and attunement. The right-brain approach is an important element of growth in our students' lives. The ability to integrate this skill alongside the left brain will help us develop the whole brain and build a more creative and critical-thinking student, both inside school and out.

Left Brain + Right Brain ... Opposites Make a Good Team

In the book *A Whole New Mind: Why Right-Brainers Will Rule the Future,* Pink (2006) relates the following four findings that he believes brain research has uncovered over the past 30 years:

1. The left hemisphere controls the right side of the body; the right hemisphere controls the left side of the body. Our brains are contralateral.
2. The left hemisphere is sequential; the right hemisphere is simultaneous. The right hemisphere is the picture; the left hemisphere is the thousand words.
3. The left hemisphere specializes in text; the right hemisphere specializes in context. The left hemisphere handles *what* is said; the right hemisphere focuses on *how* it's said.
4. The left hemisphere analyzes the details; the right hemisphere synthesizes the big picture. The left focuses on categories, the right on relationships (pp. 17–23).

Again, you can see that both hemispheres are important to our day-to-day lives and interactions. Each hemisphere has its own distinct function, but when they work in harmony, we are able to think critically as well as creatively to move our ideas forward. Schools need to provide opportunities for both hemispheres to work in sync to promote a balanced approach to learning. Siegel, a leading expert in the field of right- and left-brain research, has stated, "Integrating left and right helps us make sense of our lives" (2007, p. 46). As we seek to help wounded students make sense of their lives, the need for brain integration cannot be overlooked. If we are to successfully reach and bring transformation to the lives of wounded students, we must give credence to the need for an understanding of how these students are processing their trauma.

As I present to a variety of audiences, one thing that remains constant is my emphasis on providing wounded students with opportunities to tell their stories, thus getting their wounds to the surface. Siegel has stated, "Healing from a difficult experience emerges when the left side works with the right to tell our life stories. When children learn to pay attention to and share their own stories, they can respond in healthy ways to everything from a scraped elbow to a major loss or trauma" (2011, p. 28). The stories of wounded students don't have to define them; the way they learn to process their stories will.

"Our feelings are our most genuine paths to knowledge."
—Audre Lorde

Chapter 3
Key Points

- The left part of the brain serves a very distinct purpose and can be of great benefit to problem solving and critical thinking.
- The left brain is logical, ordered, rule-oriented.
- Operating exclusively from a left-brain perspective can be a deterrent to making empathic connections with wounded students.
- If wounded students are responding emotionally (i.e. from a right-brain perspective), asking "what" questions can open the door to a less emotional, left-brain analysis that allows them to begin processing their story.
- The right brain is concerned with feelings, relationships, creativity, and emotional wellbeing. It gives us the ability to have empathy or attune to others.
- The right brain reacts with a fight or flight response in the face of danger. This is a crucial response in the face of imminent danger, but if it develops into a conditioned response, it becomes an obstacle to reasoning and learning.
- We have to understand brain integration if we are to bring transformation to the lives of wounded students.

4

Incorporate Empathy

The Impact of Empathy

Since one of an educator's major goals is to have high academic achievement for all students, one must look at how empathy plays into that desired outcome. Empathy or being empathic is becoming more widely studied for its potential benefits to student achievement, health, relationships, compassion, and the positive effects it can have on our school climates as well as our communities and society overall. As we continue seeking to understand how everything connects in order to educate the whole child and bring transformation to the lives of wounded students, we are discovering that social-emotional factors are an integral part of the learning process. Once a student starts to feel safe and secure in who they are in their environment, the academic aspect becomes easier for everyone. During my ongoing research on empathy, I have yet to find any studies finding that empathy has any negative impact on learning or the learning process. If such a study did exist, there are a multitude of studies and available literature that have shown the relevance of empathic connections to increased academic achievement and life success. Medical schools are even making the correlation and requiring emotional literacy training for their medical students, in an effort to help them better serve their future patients. Pink (2006) noted, "Today at Columbia, all second year medical students take a seminar in narrative medicine in addition to their hardcore science classes. There they learn to listen more empathically to the stories their patients tell and to 'read' those stories with greater acuity" (p. 113).

According to O'Conner (2013), "There have been research findings that suggest that teachers' empathy with their pupils has a positive impact on achievement and attitude to learning" (p. 25). Siegel (2010) suggested that empathic connections should be made through (a) eye contact, (b) tone of voice, (c) facial expressions, (d) body posture, (e) intensity of response, and (f) developing a supportive community. Bevel and Altrogge stated:

> Programs need to focus on improving learning of every student, every teacher and every administrator, on closing the achievement gap for all learners, on developing empathy for others, on accepting differences and building on the strengths and uniqueness of each individual.
>
> (2010, p. 55)

Small (2011) suggested, "Learning empathy involves mastering three essential skills: (1) Recognizing feelings in others, (2) learning to listen, and (3) expressing understanding" (p. 17). In order for this to happen, we must learn how to cultivate respectful relationships within our learning communities, both educator/student and student/student. Boutte (2008) proposed, "Teaching toward a more inclusive social order or teaching humanity means working toward reducing our peculiar ethnocentrism so we can appreciate humanity and its many dimensions" (p. 171). Cowan, Presbury, and Echterling suggested:

> A lack of sufficient and accurate empathy early in life means that a person not only is disconnected from others but also, over time, becomes disconnected from his or her own internal experiences, which can emerge later only in conflicted and ambivalent expressions.
>
> (2013, p. 58)

Empathic Connections

Creating cultures that are inclusive is extremely important in helping students to feel connected. Feeling a sense of connection satisfies a student's core longing to be safe and secure within themselves as well as their surroundings, thus decreasing a child's stress and allowing more receptiveness to learning. Gordon (2005) stated further, "The child who is in emotional pain from feeling excluded does not have the heart for learning. What happens to the child on the playground or at lunchtime can have a tremendous effect on the child's education" (p. 159).

Gordon and Green have suggested that due to the world being more globalized, and the increased use of technology, students are developing into individualized learners. We see students who do not have a chance to interact or socialize and become more isolated as a result (2008). As Gatto (2005) observed, "The term community hardly applies to the way we interact with each other. We live in networks, not communities, and everyone I know is lonely because of that. School is a major actor in this tragedy" (p. 21). As educators, we must become intentional about providing as many opportunities as possible for students to work in groups. Group work allows for the development of social skills which can provide pathways for empathic connections between peers. Online learning offers many benefits, but it detracts from the community building necessary to creating a sense of belonging. Kiraly (2011) noted, "As educators, I would venture to suggest that 'connecting' to our students is an urgent need which all teachers must prioritize and we must be innovators here too. We need to make sure that our students are connected to each other too" (p. 14). Ultimately, it's about positioning students to interact with us as well as with each other. The benefits are well-documented in regard to learning, academic success, and healthy relationships. Positioning students to attune to the needs of others is the beginning of change towards issues like bullying and students being disengaged from their learning community.

Learning Empathy

In an era of endless curriculum standards and guidelines, finding time in the school day to address emotional literacy topics can be difficult. Seaman (2012) asserted that all teachers in every content area can find moments to incorporate compassion and empathy and still not have to adjust curriculum integrity, and Maxwell and DesRoches (2010) suggested teaching a unit on empathy as early as preschool and kindergarten. They referred to this as teaching emotional understanding so children learn their own feelings, but they try to teach children to be aware of others' feelings, too. Furthermore, Hanko (2002) said that the endeavor to teach empathy could be viewed as a developmental accomplishment for not only the children, but also the educators. He stated that this is especially true for teachers since they are "the only professionals in daily contact with all children of school age, at a time when increasingly complex emotional and social factors may impede children's learning, and frequently educationally dysfunctional teaching climates threaten to impede teachers' professional capacities" (Hanko, 2002, p. 15). Hanko concludes his article with information that teachers should glean from empathy training:

1. Develop practical strategies for making children feel safe.
2 Learn to value the child and realize that many behaviors are not personal attacks.
3. Utilize different teaching techniques and understand the difference between encouragement and praise.
4. Avoid judging students; seek strengths to build on.
5. Ask enabling questions that encourage children to think through their own solutions.
6. Understand that sometimes it is not about solving a problem but recognizing underlying issues.
7. Be aware that as educators, it is not our job to fix children's problems. Sometimes the act of caring is what pays the biggest dividends for students later in life (2002).

This is a helpful checklist as districts seek to provide their educational teams with relevant professional development training geared towards emotional literacy.

Empathy can sometimes be difficult to incorporate or teach in school environments that tend to be competitive in nature. However, making teachers and students more aware of the importance of empathy and cultivating this knowledge can create school environments that have more group cohesiveness for students and teachers alike. Moreover, this is the way in which empathy can support the goals of academic achievement (Weissbourd & Jones, 2014). For the wounded student, the implications of learning empathy extend beyond academic achievement. Empathic connections begin to build a bridge for the wounded student to experiencing the trust and relationships that may not come easily but are essential to success in life. According to Gerdes, Segal, Jackson, and Mullins (2011), the benefits of teaching empathy can be countless: The result is students with the ability to understand empathy in a more refined manner when it comes to social justice, social wellbeing, or interaction with individuals. Claypool and Molnar (2011) said, "We know that for some people, developing and having empathy is seen as a necessary aspect of being in proper relationship to others, a necessary part of reducing violence in society and pursuing social justice issues" (p. 184). Empathy is perhaps one of the most fundamentally necessary attributes in our relationships, so when it is lacking, it becomes one of the biggest stumbling blocks.

Cultivating Empathy

Creating a school environment that affords continuous opportunities to be empathic will help empathy become second nature. Weissbourd and Jones (2014) claimed, "Children develop empathy when it lives and breathes in their relationships, including their relationships with teachers" (p. 46). Be deliberate in recognizing moments to be empathic with your students or for your students to be empathic with others. Sometimes, it is as simple as acknowledging the "hard" that your student is experiencing. For instance, in regard to the child whose parents are divorcing . . . acknowledge the hard: "Max, I heard your family is going through some changes. I understand change can be hard sometimes. I hope you will let me know if you need to talk or if I can help you." Obviously, this is a generalized sentiment that should be personalized for the student you are talking to. If they seem distracted, tell them you understand that. If you see tears, let them know you can arrange private space since you understand that sometimes, crying is the only thing that helps. If there is anger, offer an outlet for expressing it. I once had a high school student come to my office struggling with some intense anger over a personal situation. He was so angry that he said he was ready to trash my office. Instead of telling him not to be angry and threatening him with consequences, thus negating his very real feelings, I told him I understood why he was angry and told him that if he really felt he needed to trash my office, I had one stipulation: Don't touch the picture of my wife. That simple empathic response mixed with a little dose of humor opened the door to trust. This student did not trash my office that day, but he did discover a safe place to deescalate so that he could get back to the business of learning.

Getting to know our students and going beyond the surface attitudes or behaviors to the circumstances that may drive those things is the beginning of empathy. And sometimes imagining where our students are coming from is very different than seeing. One of my daughters took a new teaching job this past school year in a district that has students coming from some extremely impoverished situations. Her principal arranged an invaluable experience for his newly hired teachers by loading them onto a school bus for a tour of the neighborhoods in the district where their students would be coming from. My daughter said:

> I got a firsthand glimpse into some of my students' everyday lives. I gained a different perspective, realizing that some of my students would spend an hour and a half on the bus before they ever walked into my classroom, so expecting them to immediately sit down to focus would be unrealistic. I have always had the privilege of breakfast before heading to school and the availability of snacks during a break. I am sensitive to the fact that that is not the case for most of my students, and there are times they come to school hungry. I am glad my principal

gave us the opportunity to have a better understanding of where they might be coming from.

I later learned from someone in my daughter's building that many kids knew that if they needed a snack or did not have lunch, Miss Hendershott had a drawer of snacks in her room. She may not appreciate that I divulged this information, but it is a perfect example of a simple gesture making a big, empathic statement of, "I see you. I care about you. I am here for you."

It is never too early to allow children the opportunity to extend and receive empathy. We witnessed a remarkable empathic interaction between our two youngest daughters, Kendi and Kemeri. They are only six months apart, but one has been with us since shortly after birth and the other had just come home to our family from China when she had to have a major surgery at the age of two years old. I took Kendi to visit Mommy and Kemeri in the hospital, and we were surprised when Kemeri (who had to remain flat on her back in the hospital crib) became very agitated upon our arrival. She kept pointing at Kendi, and Kendi kept reaching for her. Mind you, Kemeri was still learning to verbally communicate with us since she had only been home a couple of months, and these two were still learning about what it meant to be sisters. We finally decided to allow Kendi to sit in the crib beside Kemeri. To our surprise, Kemeri was immediately comforted by her sister's presence and Kendi was content to just sit and rub her arm, which is quite a feat for a busy two-year-old. It was a good reminder never to underestimate a child's ability to feel empathy, and that sometimes empathy needs no words. The sense of connection through empathy is a powerful thing.

Awareness of the Need for Emotional Literacy

When it comes to the teaching of emotional literacy, Dolby (2013) stated, "As budgets tighten and the focus of higher education shifts toward skill-driven courses and outcomes-based competencies, and away from a broad education in the humanities and social sciences, the ability to develop a culture of empathy erodes even further" (p. 63). I completely understand if the thought of incorporating one more thing into your day is overwhelming. The demands of high stakes testing have taken up a big space in today's classroom. However, I would like to suggest that we not view emotional literacy strategies as a part of curriculum but instead as a practiced response. In a research study on empathy, Baron-Cohen developed an Empathy Quotient (EQ) scale, and revealed that science students scored lower on the Empathy Quotient scale than humanities students (2011). Teaching emotional literacy, including empathy towards students, is of global importance as it not only enhances the lives of individual students, but of society as well. According to Gordon and Letchford:

> We know that the biggest predictor of later success in life is social and emotional competency. Adults who do not possess these skills are more likely to face mental illness and addiction, incarceration, unemployment or underemployment, and other negative life consequences.
>
> (2009, p. 52)

In addition, Slote (2011) said, "If empathy also helps make us morally decent individuals, then, once again, it has a social, political, and individual significance that recent scientific studies of empathy have not really or fully honed in on" (p. 14). Gordon (2005) further stated, "It is emotional literacy that opens the door to empathy, allowing us to see situations from another's perspective and to understand their feelings" (p. 117). One could make the argument that emotional literacy should be taught at home, but again, I would like to propose we view empathy as a practiced response that is incorporated into the educational culture. A child may or may not be taught to tie their shoes at home, but even if they were, that does not mean they should only practice that skill at home. If their shoe becomes untied at school, they should take that opportunity to practice tying. Sometimes, they need a teacher to show them how to tie it. Other times, they might see a classmate struggling to tie their shoe, so they become the teacher in response to the need of another. Regardless of where children should learn to tie their shoes, the world is a safer, happier place if we all practice keeping those shoes tied.

Impact of Empathy on Bullying

Some experts in the field of emotional literacy have come to the conclusion that empathy can alleviate bullying. Gordon and Green (2008) said, "Learning to relate to the feelings of others constitutes bully-proofing from the inside out" (p. 35). Further, Szalavitz and Perry stated, "Failure to empathize is a key part of most social problems—crime, violence, war, racism, child abuse, and inequity, to name just a few" (2010, p. 4). Learning empathy should be viewed as a preventative measure, which overall is a more productive response to many problematic issues, including bullying. Too many times, the focus is on what the consequences should be in response to things like bullying and crime, but by that time, the damage has been done. We need to invest our energies into preventing injustices in the first place. Moving to an empathic level of understanding takes us away from our traditional approach of judging behavior without evaluating the root of the behavior. The interaction becomes punitive in nature and sometimes escalates or, at the very least, does not improve the behavior.

Years ago I sat through many hours of training in order to be licensed as a foster-care parent. Herschel Hargrave, an employee of the training agency who had also fostered approximately 129 children at that time, shared a very powerful insight about working with children of trauma and their behaviors that has stuck with me. He said, "Trauma is like no other experience. We cannot talk kids out of it or discipline them into appropriate behaviors. Consequences never change the person on the inside; it only takes place in relationship" (H. Hargrave, personal communication, 2010). If the goal of educators is to be transformational in the lives of their students, it is imperative to develop relationships with them as quickly as possible, teaching appropriate behaviors instead of administering consequences.

Gordon (2005) determined, "Empathy is integral to solving conflict in the family, schoolyard, boardroom, and war room. The ability to take the perspective of another person to identify commonalities through shared feelings is the best peace pill we have" (pp. xvi–xvii). According to Weissbourd and Jones:

> We can't teach children empathy as if it were just a skill, like word decoding or simple addition. The kind of empathy that is crucial to develop in children is not simply a skill or a strategy: It's born of a broad and deep sense of humanity.
>
> (2014, p. 44)

Furthermore, de Souza and McLean (2012) said, "Learning programs that focus on treating the other with kindness, respect, and dignity should raise the empathy level of the individual, mature spirituality, and reduce the incidents of bullying and violence in schools and classrooms" (p. 178). When the entire school is bought into well thought out interventions that involve various strategies inclusive of curriculum and pertinent social skills, bullying can be notably decreased (Vreeman & Carroll, 2007). Bathina (2013) stated, "Incidents of bullying and hate crimes could possibly be averted if teachers take time to actively teach empathy, respect, and tolerance in the classrooms" (p. 47). Further, Gordon and Green (2008) suggested that "the development of social and emotional competence and empathy awakens the sense of moral responsibility in children for the wellbeing of their peers" (p. 35).

The World Needs Empathy

As you can see, the importance of empathy and its role in who we are and how we connect with others has been the topic of several studies and articles. As it pertains to learning, research has shown that establishing an empathic connection with students keeps them more engaged in the educational process, which is especially critical for the wounded student. Engaging with students and being more inclusive establishes a sense of community where empathic relationships can be practiced. However, failing to establish empathic connections with students can cause feelings of isolation for them. Therefore, every caregiver/educator should be equipped with strategies to develop inclusive environments for students. Understanding the value of empathy for ourselves and others should afford the insight to suggest the validity of its important role in schools and the learning process. The interactions between educators and students and the ways students behave towards one another have the potential to create a less stressful learning environment. Additionally, the presence of empathic relationships has been shown to reduce the instances of bullying.

Take a moment to reflect on your own experience as a student. Were your connections with most teachers and classmates empathic ones? So, what will the legacy of your classroom be?

> "I've learned that people will forget what you said, people will forget what you did, but people will never forget how you made them feel."
>
> —Maya Angelou

Chapter 4
Key Points

♦ In the quest for academic success for every student, educators are becoming increasingly aware of the significance of social-emotional factors in a whole-brain approach to teaching and learning.

♦ Developing an awareness of children's core longings can decrease stress levels, cultivating feelings of safety and security where learning takes place.

♦ The ability of educators to be empathic with their students builds connections and a sense of community that in turn engages the learning process.

♦ As educators, we need to position students for empathic connections with not only ourselves, but also other students.

♦ When educators empathize with their students, they are attuning to their students' needs and circumstances, which can build relationships on a deeper level.

♦ Teaching empathy gives students an awareness of their own feelings and the feelings of others.

♦ Teaching emotional literacy does not jeopardize academic achievement but encourages a positive environment more conducive to learning.

♦ Teaching emotional literacy and incorporating empathy can have an immediate impact as well as a long-term global impact.

♦ Encouraging empathy is a preventative strategy which can decrease instances of bullying.

5

Create Community

"What should young people do with their lives today? Many things, obviously. But the most daring thing is to create stable communities in which the terrible disease of loneliness can be cured."

—Kurt Vonnegut

Based on my observations over my years as an educator, I believe that the biggest piece missing for most of our wounded youth is the sense of being a valued member of community or belonging. Feeling isolated or having the feeling that no one understands just seems to deepen the sense of hopelessness in the wounded person. There is an established culture in many schools that entails specific guidelines for fitting into what might be the first chance at experiencing community for many children. Those guidelines typically include the way you dress, behave, perform, where you live, or even the way you think. The place where you should be unconditionally accepted at an early age of development is often where young people feel the least like they belong. If children do not feel like they are accepted or belong, they will not feel safe or secure enough to question, think critically, or even make an attempt at new things for fear of further alienation.

If we are not willing to take an objective look at the attitudes, methods, and practices that may be undermining our establishment of a welcoming community, many children will eventually wear the notion that they do not fit in. Not only that, they may feel like fitting in is impossible or unattainable. These thoughts and beliefs will perpetuate as students grow into adulthood.

Vanier (1992) observed, "Many people in our world today are living deep inner pain and anguish because as children, they were not valued, welcomed, loved" (p. 14). Of course, schools are not the only place that children can experience feelings of isolation. I do not suggest schools are solely to blame, but as educators, our point of reference needs to acknowledge the breadth of our influence as a whole. Providing students with the opportunity to experience community can feel like a daunting responsibility, but it is exciting to consider the possibilities associated with a society made up of people armed with confidence in their value to that society and ability to contribute to it.

Barriers to Community

A big detractor from students feeling a part of their educational community is giving the impression of conditional acceptance. In other words, giving the impression that if students don't behave a certain way, they don't belong. On the occasions that rules are breached, the act of forgiveness that makes individuals feel unconditionally accepted is sometimes lacking. In order to build a society where everyone feels safe, secure, and accepted, it is necessary to be able to forgive and move past the mistakes that are inevitable because we are all flawed human beings. As Zahnd said, "To maintain even the most cursory level of social interaction, there must be a willingness to overlook the occasional trifling affront" (2010, p. 23). If students in our schools feel that they must attain a level of perfection to be accepted, we have already begun to fail them.

Let's think about behavior charts or progress walls for a moment. These things are widely accepted tools used in classrooms, but consider what they might accomplish that is contrary to building community: Division, stress over inadequacy, fear of failure, to name a few. For the wounded student, the overwhelming result of a public measuring stick of compliance or ability amounts to shame. Shame is a horrible feeling for anyone, but it tends to be a powerful trigger for children of trauma, serving to validate feelings of isolation and rejection.

It is possible for students to create memories from early on in life that give them the self-confidence to understand that they do not have to be perfect to be accepted, and that mistakes can be forgiven. Volf (2006) called these "sacred memories," commenting, "We receive the content of sacred memories from communities, rather than experiencing directly the events recalled therein, and these memories shape our identity not simply as individuals but as members of these communities" (p. 99).

We live in a throwaway society, but this mentality must not enter our schools. Students need to feel that we are interested in their development as a whole person with much worth and potential. Sadly, many school policies concerning behavior are punitive in nature instead of opportunities for strengthening community. In a healthy community we can view mistakes as teachable moments, giving way to opportunities for growth, accountability, and synergy. Students should not feel like they are castaways that are expendable when they do not follow the rules.

Many educators would benefit from avoiding certain attitudes or tendencies as they strive for a sense of community connection. Some of these are:

♦ Automatic responses
♦ Selective listening
♦ Being a fixer
♦ "You" statements
♦ Absolute statements
♦ Daydreaming
♦ Being right
♦ Derailing
♦ Belittling
♦ Reacting (Wardle, 2011).

These tend to be controlling actions which do not lend themselves to a student's sense of safety and security when sharing thoughts, feelings, or struggles. An engaged, open-minded listener opens the door to students being active participants in their community process.

Building Community

As social beings, we operate best when involved in relationships based in our communities and in situations where we are understood and accepted, even in our shortcomings. Empathy for one another creates a sense of safe community and inclusion where one can develop a sense of purpose or identity. Siegel (2010) said, "Our relationships involve our connection to other people in pairs, families, groups, schools, communities, and societies" (p. 267). As we seek to build the sense of community in our school cultures, we need to be deliberate in acknowledging the role that members of the extended community might serve in that development. First and foremost, the involvement of parents is essential as we seek to understand where our students are coming from and how we might best establish a connection with them. Sometimes, parents of wounded students can be tentative, for fear of judgment based on their child's struggles. Open the lines of communication with parents on the premise of teamwork, leaving all presuppositions out of the equation. I have actually begun inviting parents when I provide training for school districts. They are our partners, and it is invaluable to establish a relationship between the school and parents built on mutual respect and support. The inclusion of parents also allows sustainability into the redesigning of our school communities.

Other groups in the extended community that I have witnessed becoming valuable assets to schools are local businesses, local social service agencies, juvenile courts, colleges/universities, and churches, to name but a few. Just recently, I was invited to conduct a two-day workshop in South Carolina for a school system. The local community college and community business council recognized the link between student success, postsecondary education, and community development and wanted to invest in a palpable way by sponsoring professional development training for the educators in the local schools. This is an excellent example of partnership for the benefit of community now and in the future. Your local community may have unique organizations just waiting to be tapped into. The more people with a vested interest in bringing transformation to the lives of wounded students, the better able we are to position them to be community involved.

As we seek to inspire and develop a sense of community in our schools, it is imperative that we never lose sight of individuality. Vanier (1992) said, "Community is not uniformity. There is a danger today, in our world, to want everybody to be the same, but then we lose our uniqueness. The incredible thing about us as human beings is how unique each one of us is" (p. 43). Think of what the possibilities would be if we could connect each person's individual strengths within a community! The beginning of the possibilities is when we recognize redeeming qualities in every child, even in the ones who are struggling the most. That can be a tall order, can't it? I understand this not just on a professional level, but on a very personal level. My wife, Dardi, and I have had days where we look at each other as we are parenting children from hard places and it feels like the majority of our interactions have been corrective in nature. After just so much of that, the last thing we feel like giving energy to is finding a bright spot. But an interesting thing happens when we make the effort to focus on finding a strength to praise: That becomes the bright spot. You can instantly see it in their faces, and a positive connection is made. We can never forget that wounded children often need someone else to see in them what they cannot see in themselves. It takes time, patience, repetition, and frankly, a relentless determination to cultivate a conviction in wounded children that their worth is bigger than their wounds. Keep at it. The investment is worth it because once children begin to believe they matter, that they are significant in this world, the possibilities for transformation are endless.

> "One of the marvelous things about community is that it enables us to welcome and help people in a way we couldn't as individuals. When we pool our strength and share our work and responsibility, we can welcome many people, even those in deep distress, and perhaps help them find self-confidence and inner healing."
>
> —Jean Vanier

Chapter 5
Key Points

◆ Wounded students need to feel that they belong in their learning community early on. Feeling isolated within this community only feeds their false belief of unworthiness, which then follows them into larger communities.

◆ Provide opportunities for wounded students to interact within their community. This encourages a sense of purpose and belonging.

◆ When seeking opportunities to experience community, do not limit yourself to the inside of your school building. Seek opportunities that give students the chance to establish a sense of connection to their neighborhood communities. This invokes a sense of ownership and belonging.

◆ True community values its members, recognizing that each has special contributions to make to their community. Having a sense of belonging is critical in helping wounded students feel safe and secure enough to begin exploring their unique gifts and abilities.

6

Develop a Professional Plan

Whether I am speaking at a national conference or conducting a small workshop, everyone seems to be in agreement that we have children attending our schools that are wounded. As I mentioned in the previous chapter, the recurrent question is, "What should we do?" I wish there was a one-size-fits-all road map, but just as our students' needs and situations are unique, so are our classrooms, schools, and communities. In this chapter, I would like to highlight some strategies as starting points for developing your school culture into a transformational environment for your students.

Nine Checkpoints for Connection with Students*

#1: Never connect a student's identity to their performance, or communicate the possibility that the two are connected

Wounded students especially need to feel like they are in a reliable place to be inquisitive, make mistakes, and learn about operating within a community of peers without fear of judgment or ridicule. Schools and classrooms can sometimes be highly competitive, with the underlying tone that there are winners and losers. Our job is to protect children from this belief by not putting so much emphasis on grades or behavior that we neglect to acknowledge the potential in a student, or their worth. Students who perceive themselves as failures in the eyes of others will eventually give up on themselves, which will not help with the dropout rate. Grades, behaviors, and accomplishments can fluctuate. Providing an environment where redeeming qualities are emphasized and where unique interests, gifts, and personalities are celebrated will produce students with a healthy sense of and respect for self.

Recently, I had a conversation with a college student regarding an experience he had during his freshman year. He told me he had been humiliated by a professor in front of his entire class, which made him not want to ever return to that class. He went on to share that as the professor was preparing to hand back the tests she had given the class the day before, she expressed her disappointment in the overall grades of the class, even announcing what the lowest grade was. As she was handing the papers back, she got to this student and would not release his paper when he went to take it from her and glared at him in apparent displeasure. The student said that it was very awkward as all eyes were on him, and he was unsure of whether to pull the paper from her hand or wait until she released it. When she finally let it go, he was surprised to find that while he did not receive the grade he had hoped for, he did not have the lowest grade, which he assumed was the case by the professor's behavior when handing the tests back. However, now this student was dealing with feelings of humiliation and shame because of the perception of his performance by his classmates, based on the professor's actions. These feelings are compounded in students who are already dealing with identity issues as a result of being wounded.

So, here's the point: Was it really necessary to make the student feel any worse about the grade than he already did? Should one's identity be put at risk because it is tied to a grade? The answer is no. Shame is not a motivator; it only serves to make a person question their abilities and sense of belonging. Some students do not come to class ready to learn because they are distracted by outside turmoil in their lives, which can be reflected in poor behavior. In the case of this student, he was consistently present in class and ready to learn. Either way, shaming is not and will never be motivation to do better. Giving students the impression that your approval or acceptance of them is conditional on performance makes for a disconnection that derails potential successes in learning.

Conversely, some students will enter your classrooms already linking their performance to their worth based on past experiences. This I can speak to personally. Back in 2010, I began the daunting task of entering the classroom as the student instead of the teacher as I embarked on obtaining my doctorate. It had been a long time since I had been in that position, and I was a little unsure of my abilities in this role at this stage of my life. To be honest, my first line of thinking was the quest for high grades. You are probably thinking that I, of all people, should have known better, but at any stage of life and learning it is easy to fall victim to performance-driven thinking. Of course we should all desire to do our best, but if our best is not perfection, we should not conclude that we are not good enough or worthy. Students should not fear trying and failing; the reality is that some of life's best learning happens from trial and error, not doing everything right the very first time.

I confess that I became very frustrated in my very first class toward my doctorate. My professor was generous with the constructive criticism, but the way I was receiving it was not as a gateway to bettering myself. My focal point became fear that I was not measuring up in my performance and that my grades were going to suffer. Fortunately, my insightful professor recognized my detrimental line of thinking and gave me advice that would change the way I viewed not only her class, but every class thereafter. She said, "Keep your focus on the learning, not on the grade." Sometimes the simplest statements hold the most powerful truths, and this straightforward directive really resonated with me. One seemingly basic concept opened the door to a place of emotional freedom where my identity could be protected from the pressures of feeling as if my merit as a student would be justified only by perfection. Make no mistake, the constructive criticisms continued, but I began to view them as just that . . . constructive. I did not receive them as marks of failure, but as opportunities to grow, all because of one simple shift in thought initiated by my professor.

Truth be told, the grade I received in that first class was the lowest one out of the entire program, but that class was the one that gave me the confidence I needed as a learner to realize I was on a quest for knowledge, not for acceptance or approval based on my performance. Dr. Savage truly understood how to protect and connect the learner and the learning. I had her for two more classes and with each class, my grades improved. I do not believe this was a result of working harder or that the material becoming easier (actually, it was quite the contrary); I believe achievement is a natural result of feeling secure as a learner. Interestingly enough, when the time came to select my dissertation committee, Dr. Savage was an immediate choice. It was not at all because I thought she would deliver an easy grade. It was because I knew that she would set the bar high while also making sure I kept my focus on my research study rather than proving anything to anyone else or the fear of failure. I trusted her critiques because I knew the spirit in which they were given, which was respectful of me as a person while at the same time challenging me to put my best into a project I would take pride in once completed. I gained much knowledge through Dr. Savage's teaching, but I gained even more understanding of that knowledge through her example.

We cannot approach children of trauma using old-school methods that are based on performance. Many of them actually invoke feelings of fear, which does nothing for the wounded child except send them into a survival way of thinking that is not conducive to learning. I would encourage every educator to consider the message different motivational methods might be sending to a wounded child.

I would completely eliminate two specific common practices from the educational setting if I could. The first would be to never use food as a reward. A treat that the whole class gets to enjoy is one thing, but when only certain students "earn" food, this can be a major trigger of stress for children of trauma. There are children who have known hunger in ways that many of us could never imagine, so instead of motivating a child to behave or achieve a certain milestone, it causes a stress reaction that becomes a roadblock to the very things we are trying to achieve. Since getting a special treat at school is a fun thing, I would suggest using treats as an all-inclusive reward. For example, after a big test, give popsicles to everyone in appreciation for working hard and giving their best efforts. Even if someone didn't give their best effort, that small, inclusive gesture may encourage them to rise to the occasion next time just because of the positive association.

The second practice that should be avoided is isolation, unless it is absolutely necessary to the safety of the student or other students and staff. Many children of trauma already struggle with feelings of being left out, lonely, and/or neglected. We have a growing population of children who spent time in orphanages or other temporary care, so abandonment is a very real fear. I would suggest creating a personal space for kids who might need a break, but within the classroom. Do not use it in a punitive manner, but in a way that gives them a feeling of being in their community while choosing to regulate their behavior in a designated area. Isolation for minor offenses only serves to reinforce wounds from the past, inhibiting vital connections needed to move into a hopeful future.

> *"I've learned that fear limits you and your vision. It serves as blinders to what may be just a few steps down the road for you. The journey is valuable, but believing in your talents, your abilities, and your self-worth can empower you to walk down an even brighter path. Transforming fear into freedom— how great is that?"*
>
> —*Soledad O'Brien*

#2: Protect your students' confidentiality

Wounded students face many issues that are not only hard to deal with, but also hard to hear. When we are entrusted with insight into a wounded student's life, we need to protect that child further by honoring their confidence. Whether this information comes through information offered by parents/caregivers or the child themselves, reassurance should be given that you can be trusted to keep this information as a tool for better understanding how to best serve this student. The only reason for a breach in this confidentiality would be if there was a concern regarding a child's or other person's safety. At that time, proper protocol should be followed for involving professional help.

As the parent of wounded children, I can share with you that this is very difficult on many levels. You feel very protective of your child and their story. It doesn't feel right to divulge some of the personal things that may be having an impact on their behaviors or abilities. It is also difficult because there is the fear that someone will not be able to see the heart of the child that exists past the circumstances surrounding their wounds, or a history they have no control over. Yet my wife and I know that open communication about the challenges we face with our children gives them the best chance at being understood and met in their unique places of development. We have come to value our children's educators as trusted members of our child's circle.

> *"Trust is the glue of life. It's the most essential ingredient in effective communication. It's the foundational principle that holds all relationships."*
>
> —*Stephen Covey*

#3: Create opportunities to listen

In order to be trusted with a wounded student's story, we need to give space for hearing what they have to say. Sometimes, we are wonderful talkers but not such great listeners. As educators, we have the tendency to interrupt, correct, explain, or expand on a student's thought. It is also easy to become distracted by other things going on in the classroom—the computer, cell phone, the bell rings for a change in classes, and so on. The best-case scenario for a quality conversation is to remove yourself as much as possible from any distractions so your student has the sense that you are focused on them. If you know that your time is limited at that particular juncture, let your student know at the outset that if he/she needs more time to talk after a certain time, you will pick up where you left off a little bit later. By establishing at the outset that you really want time with them but circumstances might prevent giving them all the time they need, you can avoid giving the student the impression that you do not have time or do not care.

It is imperative that schools give consideration to how they can create a culture that evokes mindfulness towards students' needs, concerns, and any obstacles to engaging and finding success in learning. Finding time can certainly be a challenge, so I recommend that teams develop a plan for these scenarios at the outset of the school year so that people do not end up scrambling when they find themselves in the position of having to help a wounded student. Whether it is having someone available to cover a class for a bit or having access to time with the student during a planning period, come up with some creative options for generating that time.

When you are able to initiate a conversation, I would suggest that instead of asking "Why?" questions that can put a student on the defensive, you consider asking questions like "What's going on?" or "How are things going?" or "You don't seem your usual self; is there anything going on that's bothering you?" Questions that are framed more as an invitation for a student to share rather than sounding like the beginning of an interrogation or accusation are apt to give space for genuine conversation. Your next step? Stop and listen.

Our son K'Tyo's second grade teacher shared a story with us when we attended his parent–teacher conference. She had been teaching a unit on wants verses needs in class and said that a few days later, they were reviewing this as a group. She confessed that she was getting a little bit frustrated with K'Tyo because he was insistent that food and water were "wants," even after she had reminded him that they are "needs." She said she finally asked him to explain his reasoning. He said, "Everyone in Ethiopia wants food and water, but not everyone there has it." His teacher proceeded to tell us, past a lump in her throat, that she was a bit taken aback by his perspective, but glad she had taken the time to ask him. It gave her a window of insight into this little boy who spent his first four and a half years living in a different country in circumstances very different to what we know. His early life experiences have had a significant impact on how he views many things, not the least of which is the way he processes information. This interaction could have easily never happened, but his teacher took a moment to give him space to share, and created a meaningful moment of connection.

Listening takes practice, especially if a student starts down a road that is riddled with false beliefs about himself or a situation. Our instinct can be to jump in and reassure the student, but if you interject before they feel like they have been heard, it can come across as a dismissal of their feelings. And you may miss out on hearing about something that is a very real concern.

Listening is definitely a skill that I had to hone when working with wounded students. When they struggle to communicate difficulties verbally, it tends to be expressed through what appears to be obstinate behavior. For example, I once saw a student go into complete meltdown over the fact that he did not have a belt on for school and could not find one to put on. He literally shut down and was lying on the floor in the middle of the hallway, refusing to move. He had people telling him what to do (get up off the floor), he had people warning him of the consequences for his noncompliance, but it was not until a teacher sat beside him on the floor and said, "What's going on?" that the student sat up and explained that he could not do school without a belt. Unbeknownst to those looking on, this boy had been the victim of sexual abuse. For him, a belt was not just a fashionable accessory to his wardrobe but a matter of safety and security.

Obviously, there is no way to know every wound that a child carries with them and what might trigger it, but we can be intentional about making space for children to communicate. For this student, having a belt was a very real need, and the teacher was able to allow for him to convey that need. The teacher proceeded to acquire a belt for this young man and he headed off to class without further incident. Every student has a voice; every one of them needs someone to listen.

In a YouTube interview with Father Gregory Boyle, author of *Tattoos on the Heart*, Father Gregory stated that kids "can't see their way clear to transform their pain, so they continue to transmit it" (Tippett & Boyle, 2012). This is a powerful statement as we consider the importance of giving our wounded students time and space for communicating their fears, their needs, their hurts, their weaknesses, and their stumbling blocks. The willingness to listen and hear where a wounded student is coming from may just open the door to that student having hope.

> "Too often we underestimate the power of a touch, a smile, a kind word, a listening ear, an honest compliment, or the smallest act of caring, all of which have the potential to turn a life around."
>
> —Leo Buscaglia

#4: Create safe places

Some wounded students have an awareness of their triggers and the need for a safe place to deescalate themselves. Feeling trapped will, at the very least, cause a student to go into survival mode, which takes all the focus off learning. At its worst, feeling trapped will result in disruptive behavior. If a student is able to articulate what he/she needs in order to calm down, allowing accommodations within reason is an excellent avenue to establishing feelings of safety and mutual trust. I have seen some students who will ask to go sit in the assistant principal's office as a way to sort things out. However, I have seen other students come unglued at the mention of being sent to the assistant principal's office. In my years as an assistant principal, I can honestly say that I solved more issues with wounded students outside my office than in it, just because most of the students' previous experiences with being sent to the office were negative. That was just the culture of that school. Your school may have established a different view of the assistant principal's office, which I think would be great.

Brainstorming a plan and establishing the safe places within your school before the school year starts would be better than trying to figure it out in the midst of a crisis situation. Fire drills, tornado drills, and intruder drills are mandatory so that in the event of a threat to physical safety, we are prepared to respond effectively and in the best interest of our students' physical safety. The question now is how are we preparing for students who are in emotional crisis? I do not suggest that all personnel need to take on the role of counselor, but I do propose that every member of the educational team be prepared to respond to a wounded student in emotional crisis. That initial response to emotional crisis can either exacerbate the situation or bring the student in crisis some relief, while also keeping other students in close proximity to the situation safe from emotional or physical harm. Some of this goes back to the steps described above and involves recognizing that there may be extenuating circumstances, or something in a student's background that you know nothing about, and you may need to just stop and listen. Let's face it, those two things may not be at the forefront of a person's mind in the midst of a kid going ballistic with curse words and/ or dysfunctional behaviors. The kneejerk reaction can easily be to take this kind of disruption personally, especially if you have not been equipped with a practiced response ahead of time.

Dr. Terry Wardle stated, "I recommend that the caregiver emphasize the importance of a safe place where the broken person can express negative feelings, free from condemnation and judgment" (2001, p. 171). As the caregiver to wounded students in emotional crisis, it is critical for members of the educational team to be prepared ahead of time to avoid their own natural fight or flight response and instead feel equipped to offer a safe physical and emotional space for de-escalation. Wardle further stated, "Safe people are able to empathize yet not react out of their own personal involvement" (2001, p. 171).

Depending on the ages of your students and room availability, it would be ideal if there were places adjoining classrooms or supervised places outside the classroom that contain some sensory items or at the very least provide privacy. I used to keep magnetic puzzles, a Rubik's cube, and scratch paper available on my desk. Other suggestions would be play dough, a yoga ball for bouncing, or building blocks. The key is establishing the safe places ahead of time and communicating a plan with your colleagues as well as with the students who may need to utilize them. Not only does this give everyone involved a sense of empowerment in the midst of trouble, but it also gives that very critical safe space in which wounded students can be heard.

"Relational trust is built on movements of the human heart such as empathy, commitment, compassion, patience, and the capacity to forgive."

—*Parker J. Palmer*

#5: Express to your students that they are the reason you love to do what you do, be it teaching, coaching, advising, mentoring, or facilitating any number of educational or extracurricular activities

Every person in the world needs to be needed. Your wounded students are no exception, but the concept may be very foreign to a child who has experienced rejection and isolation on a regular basis. Making a sweeping statement such as, "You are the reason I love to teach!" won't cut it. Each student needs to feel like a contributing member to that sentiment in a tangible way. Take note of the child who holds the door for someone, the child who ties another's shoes, the child who picks up the scrap of paper off the floor and throws it away . . . You get the idea.

For some of your kids, it might take a more intentional effort to find that perspective. In the case of the student who always seems to be running late to school, you might choose to see a student who came to school in spite of the circumstances that keep them running behind. They could have just as easily stayed at home. In the case of the student who is falling short academically, you might choose to see their effort. Every student, regardless of their academic, social, or emotional progress, should be validated as being an important part of your school, cast, team, and so on. Developing an emotional literacy statement like this one on a regular basis allows us to be intentional about the way we are viewing and connecting with our students.

As mentioned before, we are all keenly aware of the added stresses in education today. These stresses can easily contribute to the distance between teacher and student growing ever wider. It is our personal and professional responsibility to be intentional about communicating to our students that they are our sole purpose for teaching, whether in the classroom or in an extracurricular capacity.

In your career as an educator, you are bound to witness students finally reaching certain milestones or achieving academic goals. Witnessing these moments is so much sweeter for the educator and the student if it is a connected experience. At the end of this past school year, it was evident that my daughter Kaya's first grade teacher, Mrs. Myers, made this kind of connection at a deep level with her students. During Teacher Appreciation Week, the parent–teacher organization at our children's school gave every student a paper to fill out about their teachers, to be placed in a binder as a gift. Kaya wrote that her favorite thing about her teacher was that "she is loving to us."

I know that my daughter spent a great deal of time during the school year learning wonderful things from her teacher, but I find it very telling that what stands out the most is the emotional connection her teacher made with her. This is a perfect example of what it looks like to teach to the whole child. At this point I would also like to mention that Mrs. Myers was named Teacher of Year for the elementary schools in our school district. She is recognized as one of the top educators in her profession, and her connection with her students is a wonderful illustration

My name is:

Kaya

My favorite thing about my teacher is: She is Loving to us.

of the power of conveying that her students are the reason she is a teacher. In the midst of full plates and stressful standards, it is good for students and teachers alike to be reminded of the reason people become teachers in the first place.

Early in my own career, I was a teacher and coached football in a small rural high school in Ohio. We had what was called Family, Fathers, and Football Night, gathering as a team to watch Monday night football together in the school library. What I had not prepared for was Terrence.** He asked if he could sit and watch the game with me because his dad was not there. That was the beginning of a relationship that has spanned over twenty years.

Terrence was an excellent student and athlete, but he suffered from the emotional wounds of having an absent father. He was very fortunate to have a good mother who loved him, but she worked hard at two jobs to support her children, which made it difficult for her to be present for everything. Terrence shared with me that he struggled with feelings of anger and jealousy when he saw the other dads in the stands. When other kids told Terrence they wished they had his skills and abilities, he told them he would trade places with them any day because their dad was there to cheer them on.

Over the next couple of years, Terrence and I continued to build our relationship. He became comfortable asking me questions because he knew he could depend on me for honest answers and feedback.

Terrence went on to college, and I kept in touch with him as he continued to do well both in and out of the classroom. I always let him know how proud I was of him. After his junior year, Terrence's mother was having a difficult time making ends meet, so he made the difficult decision to leave school to help her out. He also got married, and my wife and I developed a good relationship with him and his wife, Kristen.**

One summer day, I received a phone call from Kristen. She said she would appreciate it if I spoke to Terrence about going back to college to finish up his degree. She felt he would listen to me, so the next time we got together, I pulled Terrence aside and encouraged him to finish what he had started—for himself, his family, and his future. I stressed the importance of having some type of degree or technical preparation to obtain work in today's world, but more importantly, I told Terrence that he had gifts that he needed to utilize for himself and others.

A year and a half later, I watched Terrence graduate from college. As he received his diploma, I was filled with great pride and admiration for the young man who had come so far through life's obstacles. Today, Terrence is a teacher in a correctional facility helping students overcome their wounds through education. He is also an assistant high school football coach. His players are some of the best in the state, and for the past few years, the team has gone undefeated and won two conference championships.

Terrence taught me that sometimes our area of greatest weakness can become our area of greatest strength. If Terrence had not encountered the obstacles he had, he may have never been motivated to become a teacher in a position to help so many others. He also taught me to always be mindful of the emotional state of my students. As Terrence's teacher and coach, had I ignored where he was coming from emotionally, had I given the impression that I was not interested, I may never have developed the kind of genuine relationship with him that spurred him on to finishing high school and college.

> "By building relations we create a source of love and personal pride and belonging that makes living in a chaotic world easier."
>
> —Susan Lieberman

#6: Provide opportunities for students to experience empathy or compassion from or for their classmates or others in their community

Teaching emotional literacy is one thing, but providing opportunities to experience it is another. Because emotional literacy is based on feelings, we must experience those feelings to understand the depth of their power. Siegel (2007) suggested, "Cultivating an experiential understanding of the mind is a direct focus of mindful awareness: We come not only to know our own minds, but to embrace our inner worlds and the minds of others with kindness and compassion" (p. xv).

Currently, I arrange internship experiences for students who are studying to become teachers. When I first began in this position, I realized that students were hearing about things like poverty, diversity, and global awareness, but the only opportunity to experience any of these things firsthand involved going abroad for their student teaching internship. However, for personal and/or financial reasons, this was not a feasible option for the majority of internship candidates. In response, I developed partnerships with other school districts across the United States in order for students to have the opportunity to experience life in different communities. Life experiences and the emotions that go with them are critical to growth and lend themselves to opportunities for giving and/or receiving empathy. It has been a privilege to hear from these students about what they see, what they hear, what they learn about others, and especially what they learn about themselves. I remember one student in particular who was placed in another part of the country about 1300 miles from her family and the comfort of everything she knew. She called me at about 3:30 on a Friday afternoon after school let out for the weekend. When I answered the phone, it was obvious that she was crying and upset. She said, "Dr. Hendershott, I don't like this and it's not fair."

"What don't you like and what isn't fair?"

"I'm in the parking lot on my way home from school and I had to pull over to call you. What's not fair is that my students are poor and coming to school hungry and they have a hard time concentrating and learning because of it. Some of them are having a hard time because English isn't their first language. It just sucks because these kids are going to be taking a state test to measure their academic competencies and my teaching performance, and it's not fair because their hunger and their lack of exposure to the language and all this other stuff isn't taken into consideration."

I'll be honest. The protective "dad" side of me comes out where my students are concerned, and my initial thought was that I had placed my student in an uncomfortable situation and that I needed to get her out of there. However, after taking a step back I realized as an educator what I also had to realize as a parent: You can either try to protect those in your care from the hard realities of life, or you can position them to be prepared to face them. Really, the whole purpose of this internship program was and is to prepare future educators for the realities they will face and give opportunities to experience empathy or compassion for their students, many of whom are wounded. I told my student that I was proud of her for her ability to be empathic with regard to her students' needs and struggles and then asked her what she planned to do in response to these challenges. She informed me that the following Monday, she went back to school with a renewed sense of vision and mission for reaching her students right where they were. I was and continue to be very proud of this student because I know that she continues to impact her students by working with them on a cognitive and emotional level, even when it is hard.

Experiencing empathic connections firsthand is a far greater teacher in the transformational process than simply talking about it, whether your students are preschoolers or college interns. While you might not be sending your grade school students off to another state or country for a field experience, you can be deliberate in giving meaningful opportunities for them to experience empathy and compassion in your classrooms and even in your communities. I have seen teachers and even whole schools initiate projects in their community to help the elderly, assist their local animal shelter, reach out to the homeless, volunteer with the Special Olympics or even show up just to be the athletes' biggest fans for the day . . . Really, the possibilities are endless! This is not just community service, but is a way of creating intentional experiences that afford students real-life, meaningful understanding of emotional literacy.

> *"Our human compassion binds us the one to the other—not in pity or patronizingly, but as human beings who have learnt how to turn our common suffering into hope for the future."*
> —Nelson Mandela

#7: Find the redeeming qualities in wounded students

This has been discussed, but it is worth repeating. I know that in the midst of tough behaviors and messy days, a redeeming quality can be hard to come by, but it matters. It matters not just to the wounded student who needs uplifting, but it matters to you. Speaking genuine words of hope, encouragement, and appreciation can have a profound impact on the tone of your mood. Most of us don't think twice about thanking someone for holding a door open for us as a recognition of their thoughtfulness. What if it became second nature to recognize the redeeming qualities of others in our schools? I believe we would be creating an atmosphere very conducive to a peaceful existence.

I would like to point out that we can even find redeeming qualities in the worst situations. Let's say a student commits an offense that warrants suspension because it involves a non-negotiable (drugs, violence, weapons, etc.). Can we execute justice and still find redeeming qualities as an empathic educator? Consider that no matter what a student has done, they will eventually be coming back to school. Do we want them coming back with a sense of hope or vengeance? I would prefer hope, myself. Finding a redeeming quality does not excuse or endorse the infraction, but it does allow the wounded student to feel like they have something to build on when they return. If we inflict a sense of hopelessness, we can never expect to inspire change.

"Hope is being able to see that there is light despite all of the darkness."

—Desmond Tutu

#8: Develop an effective peer process in your classroom or building

Giving students the opportunity to work with others provides meaningful experiences in teamwork and community as well as developing social and critical thinking skills. There are two different types of peer learning: peer tutoring and peer collaboration. Damon (1984) explained, "We use peer tutoring for transmitting information and drilling special skills; peer collaboration for facilitating intellectual discovery and acquisition of basic knowledge"

(p. 331). Many educators have used peer tutoring to assist students who may need additional help from a student who is a little more confident in a certain content area than another. There are multiple benefits to peer tutoring. Students who need the help can receive individual attention, which can have some real benefits in building trust and relationships with peers. For the peer tutor, their own learning can be strengthened by transmitting information to others verbally while feeling purposeful in helping another person through sharing their knowledge.

One of my daughters is a first grade teacher. First graders are typically expected to complete nightly reading at home. (As well as having a daughter teaching first grade, we also have a daughter in first grade, so I know all about this since I am signing a reading log every night myself.) For one reason or another, several of her students do not have anyone doing their nightly reading with them. Instead of seeing opportunities for consequence, she saw the benefit of connecting her students with reading buddies from a fourth grade classroom. This gives her students the advantage of their nightly reading, and at the same time gives the older students a sense of confidence and purpose as they help someone. Allowing for students to work together also helps everyone to be engaged while you might be focusing your attentions on other students.

Peer tutoring appears on the surface to be one person assisting another, but in reality it becomes a symbiotic relationship. Wounded students could benefit from being on either side of peer tutoring with clear guidelines, expectations, and oversight to ensure a worthwhile experience. Using the parameters of students' personalities and temperaments is a good starting point for effectively pairing students.

Through the study of three major theorists of peer education, Damon derived the following:

1. Through mutual feedback and debate, peers motivate one another to abandon misconceptions and search for better solutions.
2. The experience of peer communication can help a child master social processes such as participation

and argumentation, and cognitive processes such as verification and criticism.

3. Collaboration between peers can provide a forum for discovery learning and can encourage creative thinking.

4. Peer interaction can introduce children to the process of generating ideas and solutions with equals in an atmosphere of mutual respect. This in turn can foster an orientation toward kindness and fairness in interpersonal relationships.

5. However great its educational potential, peer interaction does not best serve all developmental purposes. For example, teaching children the realities of the status quo and respect for social order is done most naturally in the context of the adult–child relation.

(1984, p. 335)

In my experiences with various educational settings, as both an educator and as a visitor, I have seen peer learning with wounded students work extremely well in some instances and fall apart at the seams in others. When working with wounded students, I believe the following considerations should be made to ensure an effective process:

♦ Communication of expectations before initiating peer learning experiences can alleviate any confusion or feelings of uncertainty, thus giving a better chance for a meaningful experience for all participants.

♦ Each participant needs to understand what empathy means so they can practice being empathic to one another's social, emotional, and academic needs.

♦ Each participant needs to acknowledge that one goal is for everyone to be equally gaining from and contributing to the process.

♦ Mutual respect is given and earned for everyone's part in the process.

♦ Each participant should understand that another goal of peer learning is sharing new perspectives between participants so that a broadened sense of self and others is obtained. No one has to feel right or wrong.

◆ Each participant in peer learning should feel empowered to express any discomfort felt by any situation (for example, when someone in the group has a false sense of authority and is exercising it with others inappropriately) to the teacher.

◆ Each participant should feel entitled to give and ask for help.

◆ No participant should be made to feel either inferior or superior to another.

◆ As classroom dynamics fluctuate and personalities are learned and observed, do not hesitate to make adjustments to student pairings.

I found over the years that keeping wounded students engaged in the classroom was beneficial, whether it was with me as their teacher or in peer learning situations. As stated in a study examining elementary and secondary outcomes of peer tutoring, "Findings suggest that peer tutoring is an effective intervention regardless of dosage, grade level, or ability status. Among students with disabilities, those with emotional and behavioral disorders benefited the most" (Bowman-Perrott, Davis, Vannest, Williams, Greenwood, & Parker, 2013, p. 39). Peer learning will need to be formulated to suit the unique makeup of your educational setting, but it is worth the endeavor as an effort to continue bridging the gap that may exist between wounded students and their learning communities.

> *"I love those connections that make this big old world feel like a little village."*
>
> —Gina Bellman

#9: Seek restorative justice as an alternative discipline approach

Restorative justice takes place when a person who has committed an offense against another person is given the chance to acknowledge their wrongdoing and rectify the situation. I have found that many students, when given the chance, will do the right thing. In the case of wounded students, they have usually become accustomed to being ushered straight into consequences instead of being invited to become an active participant in making things right. This lends itself to further anger, frustration, and no practical experience in restoring relationships. This is detrimental not only to the school community, but to the extended community as well.

Several years ago, I was the new principal for a school. On one of my first days, a seventeen-year-old student was sent to my office for cussing out a teacher. Once he sat down, I just let him sit for a bit while I took care of some paperwork. He finally said, "Well, what are you going to do to me?"

I responded, "Well, what are you going to do?"

"What do you mean?"

"Have you been taught the difference between right and wrong?"

"Yes."

"Were you right or wrong?"

"Wrong."

"Do you need another man to solve your problems?"

"No."

"Go solve your problem."

The young man got up and left my office. Later that day, I caught sight of the teacher involved in the incident making a beeline for me from down the hall in an obviously flustered state.

"What in the world did you do to that kid?"

"What do you mean?"

"What did you do? I've never in all my years of teaching ever had a student come and apologize to me."

I shared this story in my first book, *Reaching the Wounded Student*, but it is one worth repeating. Learning to repair relationships is a necessary life skill that no consequence will teach, but people must be given the opportunity to own up to their mistakes in order to ask for, and receive, forgiveness. Consequences rarely ever result in changed behavior.

Amstutz and Mullet (2005) give the following key goals for restorative justice:

- ◆ To understand the harm and develop empathy for both the harmed and the harmer.
- ◆ To listen and respond to the needs of the person harmed and the person who harmed.
- ◆ To encourage accountability and responsibility through personal reflection with a collaborative planning process.
- ◆ To reintegrate the harmer (and, if necessary, the harmed) into the community as valuable, contributing members.
- ◆ To create caring climates to support healthy communities.
- ◆ To change the system when it contributes to the harm.

(p. 10)

As you know, most school protocols for disciplinary issues are based on the rules set forth in a school handbook that has been board approved. Rules are a necessary part of school culture. They set parameters and clear expectations so that everyone feels safe and secure within the learning environment, keeping a sense of order. The stated consequences in response to rule infractions are great guidelines that give a level of consistency, but many of the rules and ensuing consequences do not involve measures for reconciling the resulting rift in school culture or the people involved in the violation. The expectation is that the student will correlate the infraction of school policy with the punishment, and will avoid making the same mistake again so as not to risk repeated consequences. Fair, consistent consequences can be a useful tool, but they do not always provide a student with a conscious link to the person(s) who was offended and how they may have made them feel. I believe this to be an extremely important factor to address in the case of bullying, student–student offenses, and student–school personnel offenses because instead of going straight from offense to consequence, we are now allowing for a teachable moment and hopefully, the repairing of relationships. Encouraging this type of empathic interaction is beneficial for maintaining an emotionally healthy school culture and attaining the goals for restorative justice as stated above.

Restorative justice could have major implications in reaching wounded students. Wounded students are typically in a survival state of mind, not giving thought to the feelings of others or having experience with how to maintain healthy relationships with peers or their educators. Without the restorative justice component being utilized, wounded students are not learning how to rebuild relationships. Since it has already been established that students who feel connected are more likely to not only stay in school, but also to find success in school, we must incorporate measures like restorative justice as a way for students to avoid further disconnect.

In no way do I propose that your school should begin dismantling its current policies and procedures regarding behavior and rule violations. Hopkins stated:

> Often restorative practices build on the initiatives already in place in a school and can be seen as a natural development of where many schools are already or are moving towards. The approach dovetails nicely with developments in Active Citizenship and the commitment by many schools to the Healthy Schools program, which emphasize creative conflict management as part of a healthy school.
>
> (2002, p. 146)

It is absolutely alright to still have high expectations for proper behavior, boundaries, and respectful interactions to ensure safe school learning communities for students and educators alike. Restorative justice is about positioning students to learn from their mistakes on a relational level within their school communities, giving a sense of ownership and empowerment for righting wrongs. Proponents of restorative justice Morrison and Ahmed (2006) surmised, "To this end, it seeks social and emotional resolution that affords healing, reparation, and reintegration, which in turn ameliorates efforts to prevent further harm. As such, restorative justice has much to offer both individuals and communities" (p. 210). In my estimation, restorative justice has the potential to be a win-win in the quest to bring transformation to the lives of wounded students.

> *"The truth is, unless you let go, unless you forgive yourself, unless you forgive the situation, unless you realize that the situation is over, you cannot move forward."*
>
> —*Steve Maraboli*

Notes

* Elements of these nine steps were developed in collaboration with Dr. Terry Wardle.
** Names changed for privacy.

Chapter 6
Key Points

◆ Developing a professional plan will help you understand, reach, and bring transformation to the lives of your wounded students.

◆ Nine checkpoints for connection with students:

 ✓ Never connect a student's identity to their performance, or communicate the possibility that the two are connected.

 ✓ Protect your students' confidentiality.

 ✓ Create opportunities to listen.

 ✓ Create safe places.

 ✓ Express to your students that they are the reason you love to do what you do, be it teaching, coaching, advising, mentoring, or facilitating any number of educational or extracurricular activities.

 ✓ Provide opportunities for students to experience empathy or compassion from or for their classmates or others in their community.

 ✓ Find the redeeming qualities in wounded students.

 ✓ Develop an effective peer process in your classroom or building.

 ✓ Seek restorative justice as an alternative discipline approach.

◆ The key to developing an effective professional road map is to adjust it to fit the unique circumstances of your own school, classroom, or community.

7

Develop a Personal Plan

As educators, it is easy to constantly be focused outward to the needs of our students, the needs of our schools, and the needs of the people important in our lives. The purpose of this chapter is to serve as a reminder that as we seek to be transformational and attentive, we need to be introspective in order to be influential in the lives of others. Some of you may be reading this and thinking this is all fundamental stuff. Exactly! I had an educational professional come to me in tears after a training once and say, "I learned all of this a long time ago, but it is so easy to lose sight of in the midst of all the other demands." I am not looking to reinvent the wheel but to remind you of an important part of the educational equation . . . You.

Nine Points of Personal Consideration*

#1: Make sure your own identity is secure

As we attempt to reach wounded students and help them in identifying the false beliefs they carry about themselves, we must periodically take our own personal inventory. What is our identity linked to? The reason I say that you need to ask yourself this periodically is because one harsh criticism or one rough moment can sabotage even the most grounded individual. We can find ourselves operating from a point of defensiveness and/ or self-doubt before we know it if false beliefs resulting from past traumatic experiences in our own lives are left unchecked.

It is imperative that our identities are linked to the truth, not to things that are fleeting.

> *"To understand the depth of our own wounds, we each must learn the language of our own heart."*
>
> —Don Colbert, M.D.

#2: Identify your own triggers

We have talked about being aware of the triggers of wounded children, but we must also recognize our own. I am a people-pleaser and like to be liked, which can set me up for a whole barrage of triggering instances when working with wounded children. I have been cussed at, blistered with derogatory names, and even flipped off over the years. Words (and sign language) can be weapons of destruction equivalent to a toddler wielding a wiffle ball bat, but the difference is that the buckled-over result of the toddler's infraction makes for good TV comedy, whereas disrespectful behavior can cause a rift in a relationship. I had to get to a point where I could find the humor in what initially felt like deliberate attacks on me as a person, recognizing that in most instances, I was just the tangible presence that represented the reality behind a student's anger. Oftentimes, a student's anger is more about their own feelings of being discounted or disrespected. Once I was able to consistently respond with an attitude of "It's not about me," it became much easier to get to the root of situations and alleviated a whole lot of strife in my mind.

> *"Every time you are able to find some humor in a situation, you win."*
>
> —Unknown

#3: Recognize your power as a person of authority

Sometimes, children of trauma are wounded because a caregiver or other person of authority in their lives misused their power or their influence. As educators, we have opportunities to respond to the results of a variety of situations daily, and can do so in a constructive or a destructive manner. Even the student with the toughest exterior and behavior is vulnerable to our actions and words. We have to be mindful that our actions and/or words can serve to further validate a wounded student's false beliefs, inflict a new source of insecurity, or give them a sense of rejection. Conversely, encouraging words can serve to build students up, making them feel like their very existence matters in your eyes. We cannot be indifferent to the power of our presence in the lives of our students. There really is no middle ground on this; our attitudes and responses to our students are a matter of choice.

It is worth noting at this point that while you need to recognize yourself as a person of authority, you should not be surprised if a wounded student does everything in their power to deny that position of authority through attitude and/or action. As I mentioned in the last checkpoint, I have experienced this kind of denial of authority in some pretty colorful ways. You must remember that if a wounded child is denying your authority, it probably has nothing to do with you and everything to do with a similarity you have to a person in authority who abused their power with this child. Press on. Trust towards persons of authority can be reestablished through your diligence, but it may only happen in small increments. It is a trust worth pursuing in the hopes that this child will be open to future positive influences and interactions with authority figures who, like yourself, are invested in working towards transformation in that child's life.

> *"Think twice before you speak, because your words and influence will plant the seed of either success or failure in the mind of another."*
>
> —*Napoleon Hill*

#4: Take care of yourself; know the signs of compassion fatigue

The ability to care for others who are hurting or emotionally disconnected can be exhausting for the teacher or caregiver. The incidence of compassion fatigue was originally associated with medical and mental health professionals, but new research is making the correlation between compassion fatigue and educators or caregivers of traumatized youth. Compassion fatigue crosses many professions that involve working with people in need. According to Figley (2002), "The very act of being compassionate and empathic extracts a cost under most circumstances. In our effort to view the world from the perspective of the suffering, we suffer. The meaning of compassion is to bear suffering" (p. 1434). Compassion fatigue and burnout are closely related, both associated with a sense of depletion. The primary difference is based on the driving force behind the feelings. Burnout typically stems from conflict or dissatisfaction in the workplace, while compassion fatigue emerges from relational connections with those being cared for. Generally, the response to burnout is withdrawal, while those experiencing compassion fatigue tend to keep giving of themselves (Boyle, 2011). I would venture to say that every person working with wounded children will have an encounter with compassion fatigue at some point. It is not about avoiding it, but learning how to cope with it through finding a healthy balance between our emotional, physical, and intellectual selves. Everyone's strategies will differ based on personality, but you can start with a few basic questions:

- ◆ Do I have a support system in place where I can confide feelings of depletion and brainstorm constructive interventions? This support system could include colleagues, administrators, and mentors, to name a few.
- ◆ Am I taking care of myself physically? This might be an obvious one, but I have found that in my busyness and effort to meet the needs of others, it is easy to find myself skipping lunch, neglecting some time for decompressing through exercise, or losing sleep over difficult circumstances. For me, being hungry, stressed, tired, or any combination thereof is a recipe for trouble.
- ◆ Do you feed your inner learner? Ongoing training to enhance your delivery of knowledge to your students is a great thing, but I would suggest that you balance that with literature and professional development

offerings that are designed to refresh and inspire the mind and spirit of an educator.

"Self-compassion is simply the same kindness to ourselves that we would give to others."
—Christopher Germer

I believe that it is not only important for individuals to recognize the possibility of compassion fatigue in themselves, but also for educational teams to acknowledge the need for productive discussions about circumstances or frustrations that can lead to instances of compassion fatigue. It is important to acknowledge each other's needs while we tend to the needs of our students. We should consciously create a community of educators that lends support, understanding, and even suggestions based on previous personal experiences, when appropriate, to one another. Compassion fatigue left unchecked can only serve to create feelings of disconnect amidst the team as a whole, while open communication can open the door to empathic community.

Sadly, there are times when whole classrooms or even schools experience a traumatic event. It is in these times that having a solid foundation of open communication among colleagues about struggles will enable the team to hold each other up to face the adversity. One of the worst times in my life as an educator was when one of the students at our high school was killed in a car accident. So many of us at the school knew her well, and everyone was devastated by the news of her death. I was an assistant principal, so the stream of distraught students coming in and out of my office and that of the guidance counselor was continuous. Students could be seen seeking comfort from teachers at any given moment, and everyone was freely giving of themselves in the midst of their own grief. What failed to happen was empathic community for the team. Instead of our educational team coming together to endure a crisis we shared in, we withdrew to our separate corners—which, to be honest, was pretty indicative of the divisive culture that existed at this school. It was an awful thing to endure seemingly alone in the middle of many people. Najjar, Davis, Beck-Coon, and Doebbeling (2009) reiterated the importance of discussing how to deal with others' trauma individually or in groups because it can affect overall health or job performance. I firmly believe that not proactively promoting open dialogues about traumatic events can also adversely affect the overall school culture, contributing to greater instances of unaddressed compassion fatigue among team members.

"When you stand and share your story in an empowering way, your story will heal you and your story will heal somebody else."
—Iyanla Vanzant

#5: Know when to enact reinforcements

In our effort to connect with and be transformational in the lives of wounded students, we must also know when we need to defer to someone else. We must gauge the difference between the teachable moments that are best handled through our desire to continue developing a trusted connection with a student, and the moments where a different type of support is necessary. One important consideration is whether the student is threatening harm to self or others. If this is the case, no matter how much you have read or how much you want to help, it is best to seek people professionally trained in personal and community safety. Your administration and/or guidance counselors would be the first place to start so they can connect your student with the appropriate help. Another circumstance that requires the assistance of administration and trained professionals is when you suspect a child is being physically or emotionally harmed by others. You can be a great support for that child, but you cannot be the intervention. Check with your organization to see if there are protocols in place for different situations that arise outside your realm of preparation to ensure that you work through the proper channels in the best interest of the child and their situation.

"The strength of the team is each individual member. The strength of each member is the team."
—Phil Jackson

#6: Keep growing professionally in the area of emotional literacy

With much of the focus geared toward measuring academic standards and achievements, it can be difficult to find time for professional growth in other areas. However, just as our hope is to produce well-rounded students, we must invest in being well-rounded in our preparation to educate them. I would venture to guess that most educators have their content down pat, so why not seek information and training to enhance the ability to deliver that content and make student connections? Take a moment and reflect on your own experiences as a student. Do you have fond memories of content, or do you associate a positive learning experience directly with the teacher? This can work the other way, too. You might have an absolute aversion to certain subject matter based solely on a negative classroom experience. I would like to suggest that whatever your position is in education, you take a moment to develop a professional legacy statement. Really think about what you would want your students to remember you by. If attributes like being fair, caring, compassionate, invested, and/or inspiring come to mind, find ways to encourage those things within yourself and in your educational methodology. There are training possibilities and motivational resources, but do not discount the value in taking a reflective approach through journaling, graphing, or whatever your preferred strategy might be for visualizing your thoughts.

To assist you in your reflection, I have included the survey that was developed as the basis for my dissertation entitled *Educators' Perceptions Regarding Empathy and Its Overall Impact on the Educational Learning Process in Schools*. When the survey was initially developed, I had not narrowed the focus of my dissertation so it examines more than just the topic of empathy. For my dissertation, I focused mainly on questions 2, 9, 19, and 20 as they pertained to empathy, but for the purposes of reflection for yourself, I think the survey as a whole would be an excellent tool for provoking insight into your professional views of empathy, wounded students, and emotional literacy.

Twenty Questions on Empathy, Wounded Students, and Education

Demographic Information
Position: _____Teacher_____Administrator_____Guidance Counselor _____Other
State: _____
Area:_____Suburban ____Rural _____Urban _____Other
Gender: _____
Years of Experience:_____Grade Level(s):_____
Subject(s) Taught:_____
Highest Degree Held:

___BA/BS/BSEd/other baccalaureate degree
___MA/MS/MAT/Med/other master's degree
___EdS ___EdD/PhD/other doctoral degree

Licenses Held:

___Teaching License
___Administrative License (___Principal or ___Superintendent)
___Other School Personnel

Ethnicity:

___Hispanic/Latino OR ___Non-Hispanic/Latino

Race:

___American Indian/Alaskan
___Asian
___Black or African American
___Hawaiian/Pacific Islander
___White
___Other

In the questions that follow, please use the key below when asked "please circle one."

Key:
{7}Agree Strongly
{6}Agree Moderately
{5}Agree Slightly
{4}Neither Agree nor Disagree
{3}Disagree Slightly
{2}Disagree Moderately
{1}Disagree Strongly

1. How do you define empathy?
_____
_____
_____

2. An empathic connection between the teacher and student is essential to the learning process (please circle one).

      7   6   5   4   3   2   1

3. What are the signs you look for that might identify a student as wounded?
_____
_____
_____

4. I understand the basic concepts of brain development (please circle one).

      7   6   5   4   3   2   1

5. I understand how trauma affects behavior (please circle one).

   7   6   5   4   3   2   1

6. I am able to identify wounded students in the classroom (please circle one).

   7   6   5   4   3   2   1

7. Please provide an example of an empathic connection between a teacher and student.

_____

_____

8. As an educator, how do you approach a student who may need an empathic connection?

_____

_____

9. I believe teachers are empathic towards their students (please circle one).

   7   6   5   4   3   2   1

10. When you were in school, what percentage of teachers developed an empathic connection with you as a student? _____

11. How would you define "wounded student"?

_____

12. I understand how to work with wounded students in the school or classroom. (please circle one).

   7   6   5   4   3   2   1

13. How do you define identity?

_____

14. As an educator, I believe I am significant in the lives of my students (please circle one).

   7   6   5   4   3   2   1

15. How do you define transformation?

_____

16. I believe I can help students transform their lives through education (please circle one).

   7   6   5   4   3   2   1

17. I believe students need to have a strong identity to achieve in school and in the classroom (please circle one).

   7   6   5   4   3   2   1

18. I feel I need more training on how to better deal with wounded students in my school or classroom (please circle one).

   7   6   5   4   3   2   1

19. I feel adequately equipped as an educator to be empathic towards my students (please circle one).

   7   6   5   4   3   2   1

20. I believe that teaching empathy can have a positive effect on bullying in schools (please circle one).

   7   6   5   4   3   2   1

In your ongoing pursuit to personally grow professionally in the area of emotional literacy, some of your reflection and answers to certain survey questions could serve as a springboard to a cohesive philosophy with the educational team within your school. In other words, as you reflect on your own answers, attitudes, and experiences, how do they match up with those of your team? For instance, the first question asks how you define empathy. You will find many working definitions of empathy, so in order to be intentional about empathic relationships with your students, it is important to identify with a working definition of empathy for yourself that you can draw on when interacting with wounded students. Even more beneficial is if as a team, you establish a working definition which everyone can relate to for the sake of unity and shared vision. Szalavitz and Perry (2010) have a working definition of empathy that I particularly like: "We survive because we can love. And we love because we can empathize—that is, stand in another's shoes and care about what it feels like to be there." The act of being in someone else's shoes can be difficult for many reasons, not the least of which is that certain traumatic experiences of wounded children are unimaginable. Even if we cannot identify with being in their shoes for a specific circumstance, every one of us can draw on what if feels like to hurt. In my view, as educators we must have a commitment to keeping that working definition of empathy at the forefront of everything we do, because not being empathic to a child's circumstances leads to indifference to their suffering.

The second question asks you to rank whether an empathic connection between a teacher and student is essential to the learning process. What I have found is that the average answer is pretty high—usually around a six. But what do you believe and why? If you believe an empathic connection between a teacher and student is essential to the learning process, what steps are you taking to ensure these connections are being made? Again, developing a self-awareness is only going to make efforts to develop a shared vision with your educational team more productive because you can identify your strengths, areas that you would like to learn more about, and areas that you might question.

"If your emotional abilities aren't in hand, if you don't have self-awareness, if you are not able to handle your distressing emotions, if you can't have empathy and have effective relationships, then no matter how smart you are, you are not going to get very far."

—Daniel Goleman

#7: Find your mentor

There is a growing trend in school districts to assign a mentor to new teachers. This is a great way of making the new kid on the block feel connected to someone who can give some guidance. It can be a source of encouragement and lend support. This type of mentor can be invaluable, but it is more than likely that they are still on a journey of becoming the best educator they can be, too. What I would like to propose is that you find your big-picture mentor; the educator that you want to be when you "grow up." To piggyback off of #6 with a little twist, think back to one of your favorite teachers. There you will find one mentor.

In the seventh grade, my English teacher was Mr. Kowalka. Money was really tight for my family, so my mom sewed a lot of our shirts for school. During the holidays, all of my classmates were discussing what gifts they would be giving to the teachers. I knew I wanted to give gifts, too, but I wasn't sure how that was going to happen. My mom took some of the leftover material she had and made ties to give to my male teachers. I remember feeling a lot of trepidation about giving Mr. Kowalka a purple polka dot tie that was made with a lot of heart but (by the standards of a seventh-grade boy) was kind of hideous in appearance. As expected, Mr. Kowalka gushed over every gift he received, including the purple polka dot tie. What I did not expect was to walk into class the next day to find Mr. Kowalka wearing that purple polka tie with pride. You might not think such a gesture would matter; I'm not even sure I realized it would matter, but it did. It made me feel like I was accepted, appreciated, and that my feelings mattered. That English class became one of my favorite classes, where I achieved probably the best grades I would encounter in middle school, but probably the greatest lessons I took away from it had nothing to do with the subject matter. I have thought back on my interactions with Mr. Kowalka often as I have aspired to make an impact on the students I cross paths with, and I am thankful that I just recently had the opportunity to tell him so when I ran into him in the doughnut line at the bakery. So, again, think back to some of your favorite teachers along the way and there you will find some mentors. How will you model the characteristics of the best teachers you ever had?

Another type of mentor is someone who not only models behavior but also provides knowledge and understanding of the way to do something. I had the traditional training that every teacher typically receives from basic behavior management courses, but I knew that I needed something more for dealing with the students coming into my school broken and with no sense of direction. The most immediate source of information and advice came from the school guidance counselors, who could share knowledge and resources, including some conferences and training that would be beneficial; but even conferences and training were somewhat limited in their offerings with regard to emotional literacy. As I continued exploring information, I found a couple of authors who have had a great impact on my understanding of emotional literacy. One author whose books and articles have been extremely helpful to me as an educator is Mary Gordon. *Roots of Empathy: Changing the World Child by Child* (Gordon & Green, 2008) is an incredible read for anyone in education who is looking to be innovative and creative in studying and devising how empathy programs can be incorporated into schools, having an amazing influence on the lives of students as well as the overall school culture. I have no connection to Mary Gordon or her not-for-profit organization Roots of Empathy and have never heard her speak, but I find her ideas brilliant and inspiring, which makes her a mentor to my work.

Another author that I am partial to is Dr. Daniel Siegel. Dr. Siegel is a clinical professor of psychiatry at UCLA School of Medicine and the executive director of the Mindsight Institute. To date, I believe he has thirteen books and several research articles published on topics such as trauma, mindfulness, the whole brain, neurobiology, parenting, discipline, and emotions. These have deepened my level of understanding about how the mind of a child operates and learns. Some of his books are co-authored with other experts in their respective fields. Two of my favorite books are *The Whole Brain Child: 12 Revolutionary Strategies to Nurture Your Child's Developing Mind* (co-authored with Tina Payne Bryson, Ph.D.) (2011) and *Brainstorm: The Power and Purpose of the Teenage Brain* (2014). These books have been instrumental in my learning and research, so again, while I have never met Dr. Siegel or heard him speak, he can also be considered as one of my mentors.

While previous experiences, books, and online resources are invaluable as mentoring agents, there really is nothing like having a tangible relationship with someone who can provide insight into working with wounded children face to face. As I mentioned previously in this book, some possibilities in your community might include social workers, counselors, mental health professionals, and so forth. I have met with various people from these fields, sometimes in their offices and sometimes in mine, to glean from their expertise in working with wounded youth. I have found them to be very excited that people in education are focusing efforts on reaching the marginalized student population and more than willing to be of assistance. In my estimation, if we continue to seek mentors and share knowledge, we can only become a stronger community of educators and caregivers equipped to transform the lives of wounded children.

> *"When you encourage others, you in the process are encouraged because you're making a commitment and difference in that person's life. Encouragement really does make a difference."*
> —*Zig Ziglar*

#8: Be courageous in your creativity

People ask me all the time, "What should we do?" Hear what I am saying to you right now: There is no absolute right or wrong answer, and what works for one organization may completely flop for another. But don't let that keep you from trying something—anything—that encourages transformation, be it in your classroom, your building, or even out in your community. If it's an idea for a little tweak, try it. If it's an idea for something on a grander scale, start taking the steps to making it happen. Either way, there is no way to know if your idea will go anywhere if you don't start somewhere.

Mr. Chuck Benway and Mr. Ben Spieldenner, two teachers at a nearby high school, teamed up several years back in their desire to try to alleviate some of the drama happening in the lunch room. They decided the best way to make that happen would be to find something everyone had in common. Everybody has a birthday, and even if your birthday falls on a nonschool day, another day could be designated to celebrate. So, the Birthday Bunch was born. As you can imagine, two teachers cooking up waffles and leading choruses of "Happy Birthday" got more than a few looks cross-ways, but over time their antics created a more relaxed atmosphere for lunch. Today, the Birthday Bunch has evolved into the Lunch Bunch, and while they still celebrate birthdays, there are now many other silly shenanigans going on to keep people laughing and engaged in their community. What began as an out-of-the-box idea is now a successful program that other schools have begun to emulate, all because two teachers saw a need and had the courage to act on it, even at the risk of possible failure.

I received this letter a few years ago (2012, to be exact) from a representative of a school district I had provided professional development training for:

Dr. Hendershott,
I know that sometimes we don't always hear about the successes of our work and I wanted to let you know of one of yours at our high school.

A few years ago, you came to speak at our school. For years I had been feeling the same things you had been feeling and that you put into your book. You put a name to it and I received your book, read it and then attended your conference. In my classroom, I had been putting to practice many of the things you discuss, but I wanted the message to be heard throughout the school. It was not received well by many of our staff in the "big picture" sense and many felt we were giving kids excuses to fail. It took two years, but finally many have started to understand some of the problems that students have that are not choices and as such, are not excuses. Last month we (the school climate committee) initiated a freshmen mentoring program and had 40 teachers choose to be mentors. This is a huge success for our high school. We are in the initial stages, but the bottom line is that we are targeting freshmen with the early warning signs of failing two or more freshmen classes and having an attendance problem. We are hoping for success in forming relationships with these 40 over the next year and looking to see if we can get them successfully into the sophomore year and ultimately to graduation.

I designed a mentoring handbook that is the basis of our program at this point and I have attached it for you to review. The guiding principles came from your book and the speakers at the conference. I want to thank you for coming to our high school and planting the seed. My hope is that we will move toward a discipline system based upon restorative justice, use more community service and at some point implement a peer mediation program that my class has designed and wants to have at our high school. Thank you so much for sharing your work and inspiring me to be a better teacher.

Julie**

P.S. Today I had a junior student hand me a note saying that I was the first person in her life that ever made her feel like she mattered. That note made me feel like sharing these thoughts with you. Thanks again.

Obviously, the two illustrations above are on a fairly large scale, but transformational creativity should not be associated only with large scale projects. I have seen a great many educators embrace what on the surface could present as challenging circumstances, seeing them instead as opportunities for growth that no text book can provide for students, right there in their classrooms.

When one of our daughters was in the third grade, I was so impressed by the model her teacher, Mrs. Smith,** used in her classroom. She referred to their classroom as the Town of Smithboro, and she promoted a concept of an integrated community for her students. Many ideas for their "town" were student-led, which gave the students a voice as well as a sense of ownership.

This particular year also happened to be the first year that multi-handicapped students attended the school, and a boy named Jacob** would become a member of the Town of Smithboro. The challenge? Jacob had cerebral palsy, was wheelchair bound, and could hear but could not speak. When Jacob's special education teacher introduced him to the class, she explained all of this and answered any questions the children had. She had also asked Mrs. Smith if she could teach the class some basic sign language to encourage communication with Jacob so that he did not feel isolated. The students got to meet with the special education teacher a couple times a week to practice signing different songs and poems. Our daughter remembers that they not only learned some basic sign language, but also began taking the initiative to learn new signs themselves and even learned to sign the national anthem as a surprise for Jacob's teacher's birthday, which made her cry.

Learning sign language was just a small part of the story. The children in the Town of Smithboro took it upon themselves to assign helpers each day for Jacob. Every member of their community was actively involved: once when Jacob was asked who in the classroom was his friend, he pointed to every one of his classmates with a smile. They had become his advocates, his protectors, and most importantly, his friends.

For many children, this was their first experience with someone who had different abilities. Mrs. Smith took the unique situation put before her and gave space for her students to build community, experience empathy, and work collaboratively and creatively, which I know has had a lasting impact on those students.

These are just a couple of examples of educators who were courageous in their endeavors to develop new programming and opportunities based on the needs of the student populations in their respective schools and classrooms.

As I have traveled around the country speaking and providing professional development, there have been those who say something along the lines of, "I get what you are saying. There are so many wounded kids struggling in my school. But tell me what to do." As I mentioned above, I can't. What I speak to is meant to bring an understanding of wounded students, a recognition that we need to do certain things differently sometimes, and then encourage, equip, and empower you to think outside the proverbial box to meet the needs of the children in your classrooms and schools.

My wife does this thing when the littlest girls begin getting whiney: She stops what she is doing and invites them to sing a song, and for whatever reason they buy into it and life is happy again. Mind you, my littlest girls are five. Now, I am convinced beyond a shadow of a doubt that if my wife attempted this intervention when one of our older children was in a foul mood, the results would be way less than awesome and could even make the situation worse, which is exactly the point. Just as my wife knows how to meet our children where they are, based on their ages, the situation, and their personalities, only you and your educational team know the unique needs of the students in your individual classrooms and the population of students within your school. What works in one classroom or building is not going to fly in another. For me to offer a cookie cutter solution would not only be ineffective and inappropriate, but would also stifle the amazing creativity of educational professionals like yourself. Every one of us has strengths, and the way we get creative with our expertise is what helps define us as a valuable team member and difference maker in the lives of wounded students.

"Acts of bravery don't always take place on battlefields. They can take place in your heart, when you have the courage to honor your character, your intellect, your inclinations, and

yes, your soul by listening to its clean, clear voice of direction instead of following the muddied messages of a timid world."
　　　　　　　　　　　　　　　　　　　—*Anna Quindlen*

#9: Be ready to step into their stories

Every person in this world has an unfolding story, and as an educator you will have an opportunity to know and be part of many stories. Some of the knowing involved with others' stories will be hard, but it can provide valuable insight to the driving force behind some of your students' behaviors. It can be so frustrating to face dysfunctional behaviors that are from chapters early in a child's story. At this juncture, we cannot rewrite those chapters; but we can redirect the behavior with a healthy response. If we can think critically through the reason behind a child's behavior, we can stay calm in the midst of a volatile situation so that we can effectively address the behavior with an empathic response. I am in no way suggesting that disruptive behaviors be ignored: I am suggesting that our frame of mind when addressing those behaviors is of paramount importance. In order to best assist the wounded children in our schools, we need to have a new outlook on our reactions to behaviors. Instead of seeing behaviors as a bad thing, we need to meet these behaviors with a new wave of compassion, mercy, and grace, viewing them as an opportunity to be a teachable moment and not an avenue to punishment. By attuning to our students' feelings, we are creating an environment of hope. However, if a behavior becomes more about me and my own frustration than recognizing the wounds surfacing from a child's story, then any type of constructive recourse will be evasive. Bringing transformation involves a willingness to not only step into your students' stories, but also to play a role that contradicts what they have come to expect in response to their struggles. Do not take on the weight of arranging the details for the rest of the child's story. You can be the author of the turning point.

"There is no greater agony than bearing an untold story inside you."
　　　　　　　　　　　　　　　　　　　—*Maya Angelou*

Notes

* Elements of these nine steps as well as the Twenty Questions on Empathy, Wounded Students, and Education Survey were developed in collaboration with Dr. Terry Wardle.

** Names changed for privacy.

**Chapter 7
Key Points**

♦ Developing a personal plan allows educators to keep focused on their original inspiration for becoming educators and not become consumed by the challenges.

♦ Nine checkpoints for personal consideration:
- ✓ Make sure your own identity is secure.
- ✓ Identify your own triggers.
- ✓ Recognize your power as a person of authority.
- ✓ Take care of yourself; know the signs of compassion fatigue.
- ✓ Know when to enact reinforcements.
- ✓ Keep growing professionally in the area of emotional literacy.
- ✓ Find your mentor.
- ✓ Be courageous in your creativity.
- ✓ Be ready to step into their stories.

♦ Having an awareness of our own identity, needs, hopes, and abilities is both empowering and encouraging as we continue on our life journeys.

Conclusion

The thing that inspires me and gives me hope is the positive response I continue to receive about working with wounded students across the country. The response has nothing to do with my abilities as a presenter: it is because educators are recognizing the very real need to bring transformation to the lives of the wounded youth in our schools and want to take action. We can no longer be indifferent to the unique needs and challenges facing wounded students. Some of their futures will depend on our response. Foundational to being effective in our response is continued awareness and training geared towards reaching this population of students, and not being afraid to step out and try.

From the Desk of Joe Hendershott

After writing my last book, I entered into a doctoral program majoring in educational leadership studies and minoring in issues of trauma. I used this time to not only glean further information as an educator, but also to do some deep reflection about my passion for working with the wounded children in our schools. In the four years of the program, one of the most valuable things I learned about leadership came during an independent study course with Dr. Terry Wardle. His emphasis was on the premise that leadership is not about expertise, but about self-definition. Coursework and training are only valuable tools for helping others if you know who you are and what you aspire to. I have come to the conclusion that what qualifies me for working with wounded children is not based solely on my degree or title, but on my desire to listen and understand that there is a unique personhood in every student. And with regard to wounded students, what is true of them is true of me, and what is true of me is true of them. At our core, most every one of us wants to be heard, accepted, and feel a sense of connected purpose, but each of us has varied circumstances to contend with as we journey to that place. Almost all of us are wounded to a degree, but some of us are fortunate to have compassionate people there to help us up when we fall, giving us a sense of certainty that we can make it.

As educators, we cannot take an indifferent approach to empathy and pass it off as someone else's responsibility. Not making the correlation between empathy and the overall education of children will only magnify issues like bullying and emotional poverty within our schools and society. I would suggest that anyone interacting with children in schools be trained through an emotional literacy program conducted by professionals on the topic. This would be a critical first step in building a foundation for redesigning the school culture to be an empathic community of inclusion. Tapping into community resources such as social workers, school counselors, or mental healthcare professionals to assist with continued evaluation and integration of empathy within the school would be a recommended starting point to ensure sustainability of the redesign. Sending representatives from the school to attend conferences that offer sessions involving emotional literacy topics would be another way to stay abreast of current trends and research. In addition, I believe every student should have the opportunity to understand and feel empathy through education and experiential learning. Educating the whole child is an educator's ultimate responsibility.

Learning never came easy for me, and I am certain I frustrated more than a few of my teachers. I know what it feels like to be discouraged, but what I remember most are the few along the way who made me feel like I mattered and encouraged me to have hope in my goals and dreams when I struggled to do that myself. John Steinbeck once said, "Three real teachers in a lifetime is the very best of luck. I have come to believe that a great teacher is a great artist and that there are as few as there are any other great artists. Teaching might even be the greatest of the arts since the medium is the human mind and spirit." I was blessed to have had the best of luck as I encountered *five* teachers along the way who modeled what it looks like to make a transformational difference in the lives of the students they crossed paths with. The work I do is a reflection of them.

As educators, we must embrace the fact that we possess an amazing power to bring transformation into the lives of wounded students through understanding, empathy, compassion, and grace if we can establish within ourselves the desire to see every child as an unfinished portrait of potential. What greater gift can we give than to help students see the unfolding beauty in their personal masterpiece?

—Joe

References

Amstutz, L.S., & Mullet, J.H. (2005). *The little book of restorative discipline for schools: Teaching responsibility, creating caring climates.* Intercourse, PA: Good Books.

Baron-Cohen, S. (2011). The empathy bell curve. *Phi Kappa Phi Forum, 91*(1), 10–12.

Bathina, J. (2013). Before setting a course to learn, know thyself. *Phi Delta Kappan, 95*(1), 43–47.

Bevel, M., & Altrogge, G. (2010). Preparing future administrators and teachers: Developing empathy for individuals with disabilities. *Journal of Philosophy & History of Education, 60*, 52–56.

Boutte, G.S. (2008). Beyond the illusion of diversity: How early childhood teachers can promote social justice. *The Social Studies, 99*(4), 165–173.

Bowman-Perrott, L., Davis, H., Vannest, K., Williams, L., Greenwood, C., & Parker, R. (2013). Academic benefits of peer tutoring: A meta-analytic review of single-case research. *School Psychology Review*, 39–55.

Boyle, D. (2011). Countering compassion fatigue: A requisite nursing agenda. *The Online Journal of Issues in Nursing, 16*(1), 1–8.

Boyle, G. (2010). *Tattoos on the heart: The power of boundless compassion.* New York, NY: Free Press.

Brown, M.E., & Trevino, L.K., (2006). Ethical leadership: A review and future directions. *The Leadership Quarterly, 17*, 595–616.

Claypool, T., & Molnar, T. (2011). Empathy and ethics: A conversation between colleagues. *Our Schools/Our Selves, 20*(2), 175–185.

Cowan, E.W., Presbury, J., & Echterling, L.G. (2013). The paradox of empathy: When empathy hurts. *Counseling Today, 55*(8), 57–61.

Damon, W. (1984). Peer education: The untapped potential. *Journal of Applied Developmental Psychology, 5*, 331–343.

de Souza, M., & McLean, K. (2012). Bullying and violence: Changing an act of disconnectedness into an act of kindness. *Pastoral Care in Education, 30*(2), 165–180.

Dolby, N. (2013). The decline of empathy and the future of liberal education. *Liberal Education, 99*(2), 60–64.

Figley, C. R. (2002). Compassion fatigue: Psychotherapists' chronic lack of self care. *Psychotherapy in Practice, 58*(11), 1433–1441. doi: 10.1002/jclp.10090

Galford, R., & Seibold Drapeau, A. (2002). *The trusted leader.* New York, NY: Simon & Schuster, Inc.

Gatto, J. T. (2005). *Dumbing us down.* Gabriola Island, BC, Canada: New Society.

Gerdes, K. E., Segal, E. A., Jackson, K. F., & Mullins, J. L. (2011). Teaching empathy: A framework rooted in social cognitive neuroscience and social justice. *Journal of Social Work Education, 41*(1), 109–131. doi:10.5175/JSWE.2011.200900085

Goleman, D. (2006). *Emotional intelligence.* New York, NY: Bantam Dell.

Gordon, M. (2005). *Roots of empathy: Changing the world child by child.* Toronto, Canada: Thomas Allen.

Gordon, M., & Green, J. (2008). Roots of empathy: Changing the world, child by child. *Education Canada, 48*(2), 34–36.

Gordon, M., & Letchford, D. (2009). Program integrity, controlled growth spell success for roots of empathy. *Education Canada, 49*(5), 52–56.

Hanko, G. (2002). Promoting empathy through the dynamics of staff development: What schools can offer their teachers as learners. *Pastoral Care in Education, 20*(2), 12–16.

Hendershott, J. (2013). *Reaching the wounded student.* Abingdon, UK: Routledge.

Hopkins, B. (2002). Restorative justice in schools. *Support for Learning, 17*(3), 144–149.

Jaffe, D. T. (1985). Self-renewal: Personal transformation following extreme trauma. *Journal of Humanistic Psychology, 25*(4), 99–124.

Jaycox, L. H., Langley, A. K., Stein, B. D., Wong, M., Sharma, P., Scott, M., & Schonlau (2009). Support for students exposed to trauma: A pilot study. *School of Mental Health, 1*, 49–60. doi: 10.10007/s12310-009-9007-8

Kiraly, S. (2011). Empathy, the new educational imperative. *ACTivATE, 23*(1), 12–14.

Kouzes, J., & Posner, B. (2006). *A leader's legacy.* San Francisco, CA: Jossey-Bass.

Little, S. G., Akin-Little, A., & Gutierrez, G. (2009). Children and traumatic events: Therapeutic techniques for psychologists working in the schools. *Psychology in the Schools, 46*(3), 199–205.

Maxwell, B., & DesRoches, S. (2010). Empathy and social-emotional learning: Pitfalls and touchstones for school-based programs. *New Directions for Child and Adolescent Development, 129*, 33–53. doi:10.1002/ed.274

Morrison, B., & Ahmed, E. (2006). Restorative justice and civil society: Emerging practice, theory, and evidence. *Journal of Social Issues, 62*(2), 209–215.

Najjar, N., Davis, L. W., Beck-Coon, K., & Doebbeling, C. C. (2009). Compassion fatigue: A review of the research to date and relevance to cancer care providers. *Journal of Health Psychology, 14*(2), 267–277.

National Child Traumatic Stress Network Schools Committee. (October 2008). *Child trauma toolkit for educators*. Los Angeles, CA & Durham, NC: National Center for Child Traumatic Stress.

Northouse, P. G. (2007). *Leadership theory and practice*. Thousand Oaks, CA: Sage Publications.

O'Connor, A. (2013). All about . . . Empathy. *Nursery World, 112*(4319), 21–25.

O'Neill, L., Guenette, F., & Kitchenham, A. (2010). 'Am I safe here and do you like me?' understanding complex trauma and attachment disruption in the classroom. *British Journal of Special Education, 37*(4), 190–197. doi: 10.1111/j.1467-8578. 2010.00477.x

Paull, S. (2015). Landmark lawsuit filed in California to make trauma-informed practices mandatory for all public schools. Retrieved 2015 from http://acestoohigh.com/2015/05/18/landmark-lawsuit-filed-to-make-trauma-informed-practices-mandatory-for-all-public-schools/

Pink, D. H. (2006). *A whole new mind: Why right brainers will rule the future*. New York, NY: Riverhead Books.

Scaer, R. (2005). *The trauma spectrum: Hidden wounds and human resiliency*. New York, NY: W.W. Norton & Company.

Seaman, M. (2012). Learn how to foster empathy within your curriculum to increase the emotional intelligence of middle schoolers. *Education Digest, 78*(1), 24–28.

Sergiovanni, T. (1994). *Building community in schools.* San Francisco, CA: Jossey-Bass.

Siegel, D. J. (2007). *The mindful brain.* New York, NY: W.W. Norton & Company.

Siegel, D. J. (2010). *Mindsight: The new science of personal transformation.* New York, NY: Bantam Books.

Siegel, D. J. (2014). *Brainstorm: The power and purpose of the teenage brain.* New York, NY: TarcherPenguin.

Siegel, D. J., & Bryson, T. P. (2011). *The whole brain child.* New York, NY: Delacorte Press.

Slote, M. (2011). The philosophy of empathy. *Phi Kappa Phi Forum, 91*(1), 13–15.

Small, G. (2011). Doctor's order: Learn empathy. *Phi Kappa Phi Forum, 91*(1), 16–17.

Stetser, M. C., & Stillwell, R. (2014). *Public high school four-year on-time graduation rates and event dropout rates: School years 2010–11 and 2011–12.* U.S. Department of Education. Washington, DC: National Center for Education Statistics. Retrieved 2014, from http://nces.ed.gov/pubsearch

Szalavitz, M., & Perry, B. D. (2010). *Born for love: Why empathy is essential—and endangered.* New York, NY: HarperCollins.

Thompson, L. L. (2008). *Organizational behavior today.* Upper Saddle River, NJ: Pearson Education, Inc.

Tippett, K., & Boyle, Father G. (2012). Krista Tippett with Father Greg Boyle on turning inspiration into action [YouTube video]. Retrieved from https://www.youtube.com/watch?v=S9Mk HqlMBfc

Tishelman, A. C., Haney, P., O'Brien, J. G., & Blaustein, M. E. (2010). A framework for school-based psychological evaluations: Utilizing a 'trauma lens'. *Journal of Child & Adolescent Trauma, 3,* 279–302. doi: 10.1080/19361521.2010.523062

Vanier, J. (1992). *From brokenness to community.* Mahwah, NJ: Paulist Press.

Volf, M. (2006). *The end of memory.* Grand Rapids, MI: William B. Eerdmans.

Vreeman, R. C., & Carroll, A. E. (2007). A systematic review of school-based interventions to prevent bullying. *Archives of Pediatrics & Adolescent Medicine, 161,* 78–88. Retrieved from http://archpedi.jamanetwork.com

Wardle. T. (2001). *Healing care, healing prayer: Helping the broken find wholeness in Christ.* Orange, CA: New Leaf Books.

Wardle, T. (2007). *Strong winds and crashing waves.* Abilene, TX: Leafwood Publishers.

Wardle, T. (2011). *Healing care: The essential.* Healing Care Ministries.

Weissbourd, R., & Jones, S.M. (2014). Circles of Care. *Educational Leadership, 71*(5), 42–47.

Zahnd, B. (2010). *Unconditional: The call of Jesus to radical forgiveness.* Lake Mary, FL: Charisma House, A Strang Company.